SAVING LIVES,
LIVING THE DREAM

Short Stories by

EMTs and Paramedics

By

Nicholas J C Hoskin

&

Others

ISBN: 978-0-6152-3858-6

Published by Lulu.com

Authors Website: www.savinglives.biz

Chapters

Acknowledgements

I would like to give my thanks to all the EMTs and paramedics who contributed stories to this book. It is easy to tell your story when you are sitting in the ambulance or talking with friends at a party — it is much harder to take the time to write it down. So thank you all for taking time to share your calls and your thoughts and feelings about working on the street.

I also want to thank my friends who helped to edit all these stories, Dale Deegan, Karen Bowen, Jeff Brown, Tori Zegel, Sarah Clymer, Steve Clymer, Jenevieve Glemming, Donna Class, Shawn Stark, Linda Tate, Pamela Walker and Richard Hoskin. It is easy to think about writing a book and putting stories together — it is much different to actually do it. I could not have done it without all the help from my friends and family. And special thanks and love to my wife, Karin, who puts up with me and all my harebrained ideas.

Forward

I started in Emergency Medical Services (EMS) in 1988, volunteering with an ambulance service. I had just taken an Emergency Medical Technician (EMT) class and had knowledge of what to do in emergency medicine but no hands-on experience of how to do it. About a year later a local paid ambulance company called me up for an interview. I don't even remember applying. I went in for the interview, and they offered me a full-time position. At the time I was waiting tables and volunteering at the other local ambulance. The starting pay at the new paid ambulance was something like $3.50 an hour. It was quite a pay cut. But what the heck, I thought, this may be a good road to take.

Almost 20 years later, I am still in EMS. I have unsuccessfully tried a couple of times to get out, only to return. Looking back on my career, I feel blessed to have been involved in this type of work. I have often wondered what my life would have been like if I hadn't landed in this field of work. I think I may have been a little less jaded and less cynical, but also not as wise. Being a paramedic is a job I have both loved and hated, sometimes both at the same time. I have seen enough death and dying to last me a lifetime, but I still enjoy the big calls where life and death are on the line. I somewhat jokingly tell new EMTs and paramedics I meet that the best advice I can give them is to get out while they still can. This can be a highly stressful field, with low pay, long hours, and horrible working conditions. You may get puked on, spit on, hit, kicked, called names, be exposed to nasty diseases and see things that people shouldn't see. Even with all that, it can be an extremely satisfying job that can pull you in and make it difficult to have a "real" job.

One of the great things about this job is that there is never a shortage of stories. I decided to put this book together to share some of these stories for people who might want to be an EMT or paramedic or just for people who enjoy this type of story. Some of the stories are better written than others. Some are hard to read because of the content. Some have swear words and opinions that may annoy you, and some may slightly nauseate you. I asked the authors not to be too politically correct or restrict what they wanted to say as I wanted to present a real look at the EMTs life on the streets. I'm sure a couple of the stories will anger a few of you out there. It is not my intent to annoy or offend anyone; it is my intent to present you a glimpse into what EMTs and paramedics do.

We all have stories — the question is whether we decide to tell them and to whom. What is most interesting about stories is that any story is a personal interpretation of what happened. A good ambulance call for me, where I get to go in and do a lot of stuff and use my skills, is most likely a bad day for the patient. Or a bad call for you may be a great call for your partner. If you are considering getting into EMS or know someone who is working in the field or just like to read stories about this kind of thing, I hope that you get something out of this book.

I want to thank all the people who took the time and effort to write about their experiences. I also want to thank all the people who helped support my efforts to get this book done.

If you have a story you would like to tell, please send it to paramedicstories@yahoo.com. My hope is to gather more stories so your story can be told. All stories will be edited and possibly revised. You will be given full credit for your story. Please do not use real names as to protect the privacy of your patients.

Chapter 1

The Nuts and Bolts

By Nick Hoskin

Emergency Medical Technicians ("EMTs") and paramedics are the people who show up to take care of the sick and injured. They are trained in emergency medicine and in treating both medical illnesses and traumatic injuries. This book will focus on those individuals who work on the streets on an ambulance or a fire truck providing the medical care that is needed either at the scene or while transporting the patient to the hospital.

Upon arrival at the scene of an accident or medical emergency the EMT will provide the care that they have been trained to give. At times, this care may take place at the scene of the call and the patient may be left at home or at the scene without being taken to the hospital. Once it is determined that the patient is going to the hospital, care is done in the ambulance while en route to the emergency room.

There are several levels of emergency medical technicians. Different areas of the country use different names for these levels. NREMT (National Registry of Emergency Medical Technicians) designate four levels:

*First Responder (about 40 hours of training)
*EMT-Basic (about 110 hours of training)
*EMT-Intermediate (200-400 hours of training)
*EMT-Paramedic (1,000 or more hours of training)

EMS (emergency medical services) providers will usually have at least one of these levels of training depending on the local resources and funding available. In most situations EMTs and paramedics work together in teams. One of the members will drive the ambulance while the other attends and takes care of the patient in the back of the ambulance. During this time the EMT or paramedic is asking questions regarding medical history and pertinent medical information that may help provide information to better treat the patient. While questioning and gathering medical information there may also be a number of procedures that need to be performed. This may include starting IVs, providing oxygen or other medications, splinting or bandaging injuries and many other procedures that need to be done. Upon arrival at the hospital the emergency medical personnel will provide a report to the hospital staff. This report will include the patient's conditions, injuries, medial history, treatment and any other pertinent medical information. The ambulance crew will then prepare for the next call and clean and restock as needed.

Different areas of the country use different words or phrases when it comes to EMS. An example of this is "core-zero" or "core" versus "code"; they all mean cardiac arrest. In this book I have used the local language.

First Responders, EMT-Basic or EMT-1, are trained in basic life support. This includes basic cardiac, respiratory and traumatic emergency care.

EMT-Intermediate, or EMT-2 and EMT-3, are considered "ALS" or Advanced Life Support. They receive additional training in the use of heart monitors and defibrillators, giving fluids intravenously, advance airway procedures, plus they are able give a few medications.

EMT-Paramedic or EMT-4 allows all of the procedures of the lower levels plus they are taught to read electrocardiograms ("EKGs"), advanced airway procedures (called edotracheal intubations), and to provide more medications including narcotics for pain relief.

EMS training for First Responders, EMT-B, EMT-I and EMT-P takes place at local hospitals, community colleges, EMS academies and universities. Once training is completed continuing education is needed to maintain certification. This certification takes place at the state level. The National Registry of EMTs is a national organization that requires levels of requirements that have been adopted by many states. What the student learns is emergency care of patients in both medical and traumatic settings. This will include providing care in respiratory and cardiac emergencies, diabetic problems, controlling bleeding, splinting fractures, and childbirth, just to name a few. The student will also learn how to use emergency equipment such as splints, oxygen delivery systems, stretchers, backboards and cervical collars. Many of these programs will have hands-on training where time is spent in emergency rooms, or doing a ride-along on an ambulance.

EMS providers touch the lives of thousands of people every day. Formal training and certification is the first step to pursuing this rewarding yet challenging career. The following stories are just a taste of what life could look like while working as an EMT or paramedic. Becoming an Emergency Medical Technician may be the start of an exciting career – saving lives and making a difference.

Chapter 2

Just a Nice Guy

By Nick Hoskin

We had just started our shift at 5 a.m. My partner and I settled into our usual posting spot that is quiet and dark. We worked for an ambulance service that "posts," which means staying in your ambulance for your shift because you don't have a base (an office where you stay until you get a call). At each post we have our favorite places to park and hang out — it depends on the time of day and temperature. If it is hot, we seek out shade to help keep us cool.

We didn't have to worry about heat or shade this time of morning, just a quiet dark place to park and fall asleep, hoping to catch up on the hour or two we lose every morning we work. I already felt about six hours short of sleep this week. Just as I was situating my pillow, we got a call for a woman who was having difficulty breathing.

The call was only a few blocks away, so we arrived within a minute or two. It seemed as if it was going to be one of those days. First, we have the *way too early in the morning when we should be sleeping call*. Then we dump the cot, displacing our kit, the heart monitor, and the oxygen bottle as we try to lift our bed over the curb onto the sidewalk.

I hate early morning calls.

We walk into a private residence to find a 250-pound

9

woman sitting in a chair. She is wearing a nasal cannula that is giving her oxygen, but does not seem short of breath. It is my partner's call, so I look around the room, call the fire department to let them know they can drive the rest of the way non-emergent, and let my partner do the work.

"What seems to be the problem today, ma'am?" Barry asks.

"I think I have a fever, I feel shaky, and I possibly have a UTI (urinary tract infection)," she answers in a complete sentence, which shows me she is breathing just fine.

"How long has this been going on?" he asks.

"It started yesterday," she responds. "I took some ibuprofen to help with the fever, and after that I felt better."

"How about if we take you to the hospital to get checked out?"

"Oh heavens no, I was just hoping you had a thermometer and some ibuprofen to help me with my fever," she said emphatically.

Barry looked at me with a smile on his face. He knows how I just love these calls in the *oh my god, I can't believe we are here* kind of way. I just shake my head, roll my eyes, and tell the fire guys, who've just arrived, that I would love to let them go back to their base, but if she decides to go to the ER we would need help loading her. With the way the morning is going, I'm sure we could get her loaded up on the cot and then we'd tip her over because of her weight. We could never get her back on the cot, not to mention the paperwork we would have to fill out.

However, our patient was adamant about not going to the ER. She just wanted some ibuprofen to help with the fever. She was going to call her son to get her some ibuprofen, but she didn't want to call him so early in the morning. Barry, being the nice guy he is, asked, "Ma'am, since we are already here and it is so early, why don't we go to the store and get some for you?"

"Why, that would be wonderful of you two," she replied.

I told the fire guys they could leave and try for another half hour of sleep. They thanked us and told us what nice guys we were. It's all about the customer service.

"All I have is $2 in my wallet. I could write you a check" our patient said.

"Let us take care of this. We'll go pick up what you need and be right back," Barry said.

Walking down the sidewalk, I asked how come he was being so nice.

"I'm just helping a person who need some help. Isn't that what our job is about?" Barry replied.

My cynical side was showing and I asked, "What happens when she ODs (overdoses) on them and then sues us for giving her medication and not taking her to the hospital?"

"You have been in this business way to long. Get in the ambulance and I'll drive, go into the store, buy the ibuprofen, and drive back. You just sit there and go to sleep."

And that is what he did. The lady gave him a blank check telling him to fill it out. "I trust you," she said.

He filled in the $10 it cost him, showed her and walked out the door. Back in the ambulance, he showed it to me and tore it up.

11

"My good deed for the day" he said as he smiled.

I then realized that I am working with a truly nice guy. He got into this business because he enjoys it and he enjoys helping people. It was three months before I heard Barry swear. He is a nice guy who in some ways doesn't want to be known as a nice guy.

People like Barry help remind me that this is a good job — low pay, early mornings, crappy calls and all. This really can be a job about helping people, even in small ways. No one will know what Barry did, nor will he get credit for going that extra mile. He will probably forget about this call in a day or two.

But with this story I have passed along that good deed so you will know what a good man Barry is, and maybe that will inspire you to do the right thing.

Chapter 3

Mountain Call

By Kerry Smith

I live and work in a picturesque community in Colorado, surrounded by the majestic Rocky Mountains. It is common for the local wildlife to saunter around town as if they own it. For example, golfers often have to compete with elk and geese for room on the fairway. Every now and then, wildlife will cause an accident on the highways that initiates a 911 call. People who live here love and respect the wildlife, which helps to make the town special.

On one call I went on, an 80-year-old woman had called 911 because one of her "pet" deer that was grazing in her back yard got stuck in a fence it had tried to jump. This poor deer was hanging helplessly from a 6-foot fence with an obviously broken leg. The woman wanted help to get it unstuck. During the 911 call, the dispatcher said the caller was very upset while talking about how the deer had broken its leg, then the phone sounded as if it had been dropped to the ground. After that the dispatcher could hear only some gurgles and faint breathing.

EMS was called, and my partner and I arrived less than four minutes later to find the woman in full cardiac arrest. We went to take care of the patient, and the police went to take care of the deer. While administering medication to the woman, the report of gunfire made me jump. The police

13

officer had put the deer out of its misery. The thought that ran through my mind was that if EMS personnel were allowed to carry a sidearm, our call would have been much shorter and would probably have had the same outcome. We worked on the woman for about 20 minutes, got pulses back, and then drove her to our local hospital. She was later flown down to a larger hospital where she ended up dying three days later. Later, we learned that her husband had been taking a shower while his wife was calling 911 and dropping to the ground. He was unaware of what was transpiring in his own house and yard.

There is a program in our town that gives away the elk and deer that are killed on the highway to the locals who sign up. It is a great way to put to use these animals that are killed because of cars. I wonder if the husband was given the deer to eat?

Chapter 4

Good Call, Bad Call

By Nick Hoskin

Let me share two EMS (Emergency Medical Service) stories. I want to share two with you because I consider one good and the other not so good. But that is what it is like working on an ambulance. On some calls you get to be the hero; on other calls you wonder why they even let you drive an ambulance, let alone attend to a patient in the back.

My partner and I were enjoying a nice breakfast at the local greasy spoon. We were hanging out with one of the other crews, sipping coffee and laughing at stupid jokes.

"Paramedic One and fire, respond to 555 Cherry St. on an unconscious female, CPR in progress." The call came over our radios.

It was in the area I was covering, so it was my call.

"See you guys soon. Thanks for breakfast. We'll pay you later," I said as we rushed out of the restaurant.

My partner, Sean, jumped in the driver's seat as I looked up the address. It was a couple of miles away so it wouldn't take us long to get there. My partner had only been on the streets a few months and was still excitable. He was driving like somebody's life depended on it, which I guess it did,

15

but his speed wouldn't do us or the patient any good if we got in a crash on the way there.

"Could you slow down just a little, Sean?" I asked. Sean let off the gas pedal just a little.

We arrived on scene just before the fire department. We walked down the front walk of the patient's house. I knocked on the front door. No answer. I checked to see if the door was unlocked — it was — and I slowly opened it. I was taught to always think about scene safety even at nice houses like this. The house looked like all the other houses in the neighborhood. The yard was in good shape, the grass cut, no peeling paint on the house. Not really a place to be wary about.

"Hello, paramedics and fire department. Did you call for an ambulance?" I yelled in through the front door. No answer. This is kind of weird, I thought to myself.

I asked the firefighters if we had the right house.

"Yeah, this is the right address," the lieutenant replied.

We poked our heads through the door and yelled a little louder.

"Paramedics, fire department. Anyone here?"

No answer.

The three firefighters and my partner and I all walked into the house and started looking around.

"In the bathroom, over here, we have two down," came a call from one of the firefighters. I looked into the bathroom and saw what looked to be a mid-60s-year-old male lying on top of an 80 -something-year-old female.

"Get them both out of the bathroom," I ordered as I grabbed by pack set (radio) and told dispatch, "We need a second ambulance here."

I didn't have time to tell them why as I was already opening up the medical kit to get an ambu-bag (a device used to breath for the patient) and IV setup.

I chose to work on the man. He was younger and lying on top of the woman, and he looked a little fresher, not quite as dead. Sean and a firefighter carried the man to the middle of the sitting room floor. The two other firefighters were doing the same thing to the woman and started CPR and bagging (using an ambu-bag to breathe for the patient) her.

My partner was getting our patient hooked up to the heart monitor. Our firefighter was doing compressions, and I was bagging the patient. Once the heart monitor was on, I looked and saw that he was in V-fib (ventricular fibrillation), a heart rhythm that is non-conducive to life. I charged up the paddles to 200 joules and yelled, "Clear." Making sure that no one was touching the patient, I hit the button. Click went the heart monitor as the patient's body jumped from the voltage. His heart rhythm went into asystole (flat line) for a brief few seconds and then into a sinus rhythm. Finally, he had pulses.

He was alive again. It was time to get a patent airway, so I quickly grabbed the laryngoscope and started to intubate him (inserting a plastic tube into the trachea to help him breathe). At the same time, I saw my partner holding the guy's arm as he started an IV. My partner's hand was shaking as he did this — it was the only sign as to how pumped up he was by this call. I looked into my patient's mouth and saw the vocal cords and put the endotracheal tube right through them. I hooked up the ambu-bag and gave it a couple of squeezes while I listened over his belly to make sure the tube was in the right place. There were no sounds in his stomach (which meant that the endotracheal tube was not in the esophagus), and he had clear bilateral breath sounds. The tube was good, so I moved on to the next thing. It was time to tie the endotracheal tube down so it wouldn't come out and take a quick look at the heart monitor. It was still in a sinus rhythm. Good. My partner had the IV all hooked up and it was flowing nicely. Time to go check on the other patient.

Picking up the medical kit and taking the heart monitor, I told my partner to take care of the guy we had just worked on. Walking across the room, I got a better look at the other patient. She looked to be in her 80s, and to be blunt, she looked dead. The firefighters were doing good BLS (basic life support, or CPR), and I asked them to continue as I hooked up the monitor. The woman was in asystole but was still very warm to the touch and didn't seem like she had been down too long. I got out another endotracheal tube and intubated this patient. We had a good airway, CPR was being done, and I was ready to start an IV on her.

About this time, the two people we'd just had breakfast with showed up.

"What do you need, Nick?" Terry asked. He was the paramedic on the other ambulance.

"We have two cardiac arrests," I told him. "You should take the man over there. We shocked him once at 200 joules from a V-fib. He went back into a sinus rhythm with pulses, and as of now I'm not sure how he is doing. Plus, I need your medical kit. I'm running out of supplies."

Terry gave me his kit and took mine, with what little was left in it. The house looked like a war zone with the amount of medical trash strewn across the floor. I got back to starting an IV on the woman. Sean left the man and came over to help me.

"This guy is still in a sinus rhythm and is actually starting to buck the tube," Terry yelled across the room to me. "I'm going to give him some Versed to knock him back down."

Wow, I thought, this means the guy is doing well. I wondered if I could get anything back on the woman.

The IV had been started on the woman, and Terry and his partner were loading the man onto the gurney. I pushed one milligram of Epinephrine through the IV line, followed quickly with one milligram of Atropine. CPR was continued. By this time, Terry was en route to the ER with a firefighter in back to help him if his patient went into cardiac arrest again. After five minutes, I followed up with another milligram of Epi and a milligram of Atropine.

"Stop compressions," I directed the firefighters. "Let's see what the underlying rhythm is."

Unfortunately, we realized that the woman was still in asystole. It was time to let this person just be dead. She'd been down too long to get back any kind of life, and if we did bring her back, she would be in ICU at the hospital for a day or two and then die. I'd seen it before, and it is just a waste of money for the family. I called up the doc at the ER and explained what we had and said I wanted to terminate resuscitation on our patient.

"Sounds good to me, Nick," the doc said to me. "Go ahead and pronounce her and give me a call back if you need anything else."

"Anybody have a problem with me pronouncing this lady?" I asked Sean and the firefighters. They all shook their heads "no."

"Let's stop CPR and clean up," I said. "This place is trashed." Looking around, I realized what a messy paramedic I can be. We picked up the empty medication boxes, the plastic bags, the used syringes.

"Good job, guys," I told the firefighters. "This was a crazy call. I'll let you know what I find out."

We took one last look around and headed out the door. I took a deep breath of fresh air. That had been crazy.

We drove back to base to restock our supplies. We had to run a couple of more calls after we restocked, so it took a while to talk with Terry. I finally caught up with him a few hours later at base.

"How's our guy doing, Terry?" I asked.

"He went into the cath lab and had a couple of stents put in," Terry told me. "He's in ICU, and the doc said they expect to extubate (remove the endotracheal tube) him soon. They think he is going to have a full recovery. Good job on this one, Nick. I talked with a police officer and found out that the woman who died was our patient's mother. He went over to visit her and found her in the bathroom unconscious. He called 911 and the dispatcher told him to start CPR. He must have collapsed and had a heart attack himself. I think for him it will be a weird blessing in disguise. His mom died, but this allowed him to live."

"I love this job," Terry said as he walked out the door.

Sometimes you're the hero and sometimes you have a good call.

"Paramedic One and Fire, respond to Pines Manor at 1585

Shawnee Way on a female party that is unconscious" dispatch says over my radio.

Pines Manor is a local nursing home that we frequent quite often. On this day, my partner Barry and I had a third rider with us — an EMT student riding along to experience what he is learning in class.

"Sounds like you might have a good call, Allen," Barry told the EMT student.

"Paramedic One, fire, just an update to let you know that CPR is in progress," dispatch told us.

"Paramedic One copies," I replied.

We beat the fire department there and unloaded our stuff. We put the heart monitor and medical kit on the bed and then asked Allen, the EMT student, to grab the suction in case we needed it.

One of the nursing home employees met us at the door to show us the way in. "Just go down that hall on the left and through the doors," she told us.

Opening the double doors, we saw about five people standing around an elderly woman on the floor. No one was doing CPR.

"Hi there. What's going on this morning?" I asked.

"This is Betty. She's 67 years old. We took her in for breakfast this morning in her wheelchair. Just as we were about to serve her breakfast, she had a full seizure lasting about two minutes. She's only been at our facility about two days. As far as we know, this is a first-time seizure."

Betty was an overweight woman who was bald and looked

like she was receiving chemo for cancer. There was a little blood coming out of the right side of her mouth. She was breathing about 20 times a minute, which is normal, and was softly moaning, making a weird noise.

"What is her medical history, and what meds is she on?" I asked.

"Here is a list of her medications," one of the nurses replied. "As far as her history, she has lung cancer and hypertension. Since she only came to us a couple of days ago, we don't know a lot about her. Her usual mentation is that she is oriented to herself."

I told my partner, Barry, to get her on the monitor and asked our third rider to put Betty on some oxygen and check her blood pressure. He put the oxygen on first and started to take her blood pressure. My partner handed me a strip of paper from the heart machine that showed me she was in a tachycardic (a heart rate above 100) rhythm at a rate of about 124 beats per minute.

"The pressure I got was 180/126, but it seems like it might be higher," the third rider told me. "It was hard to get since she is moving around so much."

"Great," "I said. "Let's get her loaded up and out to the ambulance."

Our patient was acting postictal — kind of out of it. She couldn't answer any questions. Most people who have seizures will be out of it for a while. This can last from a few minutes to hours.

The woman kept grabbing at stuff and moving around. "Let's put some restraints on her so we can get some stuff done," I said.

"We were told that CPR was in progress. Did anyone do CPR?" I asked.

"No. That was my fault," said one of the orderlies. "I was told CPR was being done, so that's what I told 911, but no one has done CPR."

"We'll take her up to the hospital. Thanks for all the help," I told the staff of the nursing home.

We loaded our patient into the ambulance. The firefighters asked if we needed anything else. I told them no, and Barry jumped up front to drive us to the hospital.

"Let's go non-emergent, Barry," I told him and off we went to the hospital. Our patient seemed a little agitated and was moving around a lot. That's not unusual, and since she had her hands restrained, I didn't think it would be a problem. I had put on an automatic blood pressure cuff that would take her blood pressure automatically. It read 170/130, which is high, but since they are not always accurate, I don't entirely trust them.

"Allen, hold her arm right here and here so I can get an IV," I directed Allen, who was riding in back with me. Betty had a nice big AC (antecubital vein at the bend of her elbow) that looked like it should easily take an 18-gauge needle. It slipped right in, and I got a nice flash of blood in the chamber of the IV hub. I advanced the catheter and pulled out the needle. Allen was doing a good job of holding her arm, so things were going pretty well. I hooked up the Vacutainer, which allows me to draw blood into tubes so I can have that ready for the ER.

All this time, I was talking with Betty, and she seemed to be getting a little better although she was still moving around quite a bit. She kept trying to move her arms and head and still seemed agitated. I reached behind me to get the glucometer so I could check and see if her blood sugar was low and might be the cause of her agitation. While doing this, her other arm came free. Whoever had tied her up on that side hadn't made the restraint tight enough. I had one hand holding the IV and the other holding onto her hand that had just gotten loose.

"Barry, pull over and get back here," I yelled up front to my partner. "I need some help." Allen was still holding the arm in which I had started her IV—this was crucial so that the IV wouldn't blow. Barry flipped the emergency lights on, right in the middle of the road, and got in back to help.

Barry took some Kerlix — cloth bandaging for wrapping wounds that's also great for tying people up — and tied up her right arm. He got back up front and continued to the hospital non-emergent.

I put my last empty blood tube into the Vacutainer. No blood was coming out.

"Screw it," I thought to myself. "They can get blood at the ER."

I pulled the tourniquet off and hooked up the bag of saline. As the saline dripped in through the IV line, I saw a hematoma (swelling of tissue) develop. The IV had blown. With all the moving around, this was bound to happen.

The patient had a picc line (a more permanent IV type site for patients who are usually very sick) in the other arm, so I was not going to try to stick her again. I put a 4x4 bandage over the hole I had put in her arm and taped it down. I rechecked the blood pressure and made sure I hadn't missed anything. That's when I saw the pool of blood on the floor and all over my boot where Betty had been bleeding from the IV attempt. This call was starting to suck. She was on Coumadin, which thins the blood so that it takes longer to clot. I should have had Allen put some pressure on it for a while. Too late now. While Allen helped me clean up the bloody mess on the floor, I used the glucometer to check her blood sugar.

Traffic was heavy, and it was taking us a while to get to the ER. I was so done with this call, but we still had a couple of more miles to get to the ER. I hate calls when the patient keeps grabbing at me and can't tell me anything and there is nothing I can do for her anyway. Betty might have still been postictal — it was hard to tell because I didn't know her normal mentation (how she acts normally).

We came up to the last stoplight just before the hospital.

"Barry," I yelled up front, "get us through this light, now."

Barry turned the lights on again, tapped the siren, and we went through the red light. Barry backed the ambulance into the bay, came around to open the back doors, and pulled the cot out. Right at this moment, Betty started to seize again.

"Let's get her into the ER," I said.

The nurse who was waiting for us took a look at our patient seizing and directed us to a different room than the one we had been assigned. This hospital doesn't get too excited by things like this. We went into Room 11 and moved our patient over to the hospital bed.

Both the nurse and the doc were in the room and waiting for a patient report.

"This is Betty, 67 years old, per nursing home," I told the crowd of medical onlookers. "The patient was wheelchaired into the dining room at Pines Manor for breakfast, and before she started to eat, she had a seizure which lasted about two minutes. As far as the nursing home staff knows, she has not had seizures before. Patient has history of lung cancer and hypertension. Here is a list of the medication she is taking. She doesn't have any allergies. She started seizing right when we opened the back doors. She has a pic line on her right side. I blew the IV on her left side. Her blood sugar is 151."

The hospital crew took over. I got the face sheet (sheet of paper with patient information such as insurance, home address, and birthday) and walked out the door.

I hate calls like this. Blowing IVs, blood all over the ambulance and my boot, a call that just doesn't go very smoothly. To top it off, she seized right as we arrived at the hospital. I asked later how she was doing, and I was told that she now has some tumors in her brain.

You're only as good as your last call. Right now, I suck.

Chapter 5

Ambulance Driver

By Nick Hoskin

Montana is a beautiful state. Sparsely populated, it invokes those romantic feelings that rural states can have. It is called Big Sky Country, and once you've seen it you'll know just what that means. The sky is big there, and it seems to go on forever.

Visiting Montana when I was younger started a dream of living in this wide open frontier. It seemed like a great place to go in search of adventure and a place to enjoy the great outdoors, unbothered by a lot of people. Houses there are relatively inexpensive and the people are friendly. I've heard it described as a state that is about 10 years behind other states in growth and lifestyle. That sounded perfect — getting back to a simpler way of living.

After surfing the Web to see what jobs were available in Montana, I found it fairly easy to land a job. It may have helped that I have a lot of experience and I do well in interviews.

I drove up mid-summer to interview for a full-time paramedic position and to look at the town. I had never been to the town before and I wasn't disappointed. With a population of about 130,000, nice old houses and wide open spaces, it was beautiful. It had a hospital-based

27

ambulance system and what looked like nice equipment.

As I drove into the hospital parking lot, I noticed that there where electric outlets at all the parking spaces. It didn't take long to notice that most of the trucks and cars had electrical plugs sticking out of their front grills. Either Montanans were a lot more concerned with the environment than I thought (and hence they all drove electric cars and trucks) or this place got cold, really cold. All I could think was it must get awfully cold in a place where you have to plug in your car… but I had a love for winter so this shouldn't be a big problem.

I wore nice clothes to my interview but chose not to wear a tie because I didn't want to appear to be too much of a "city boy." Good thing, because the manager of the ambulance interviewed me, and he showed up in cut off shorts and sandals. Some of my trepidation of driving up for an interview vanished. What a great place it is where people are so laid back they show up in shorts for interviews. It was already apparent that this could be a good thing for me. After a conversation about my experience and a look around the hospital, I was asked to lift a few heavy items and demonstrate that I knew how to use a pram. I was told this was because of previous hire had hurt her back when lifting a patient, and it caused the hospital a lot of headache with the medical claims and whatnot.

The interview seemed to go well and was very casual. After the interview I changed my clothes and headed into the mountains to find a nice camping spot for the evening. It was a beautiful clear night and didn't get dark till 10:30 or so. It was amazing. This was what I wanted by living in Montana — camping that's just a short drive from town and the feeling of being in the middle of nowhere.

This seemed to be a laid back place to work and practice medicine, and a small rural town to settle down in and be part of. The stars were out and looked thick in the sky. I fell asleep dreaming of how wonderful it would be to live here.

Leaving to go home the next day, I felt like I had made a great decision to look into moving to Montana. Upon arriving back into Colorado, the roads north of Fort Collins seemed crowded and the air thick with pollution. It was a huge contrast to what I had seen in Montana. I went back to my normal job dreaming of the adventures I would have if I got hired in Montana.

About a week later, I received a call from the human resource department offering me the job. I was ecstatic! For my experience as a paramedic they were offering $12.31 an hour. I had set my limit in my mind at $15 an hour, so I was disappointed.

But it didn't take me long to justify lowering those expectations because the cost of living would be so much cheaper. Even though I'd be making less, I figured my lifestyle would be much better. I took a day or two to think about it and then asked if I could start in two to three months to give me time to sell my house and get my affairs in order. The woman from the HR department was more than helpful and said that would be fine.

It was a quick couple of months. I sold my house pretty easily and made another trip up to Montana, this time to look for a house to buy. After looking at about six houses, I found a great place. It was bigger and cheaper than the house I was selling in Colorado. This was going to be a great move. The people I had met so far were all wonderful and the town seemed even nicer as I wandered different neighborhoods and went for a couple of trail runs on the outskirts of town.

After getting my affairs in order I moved up in early October. It was fantastic weather. I experienced a few weeks of Indian summer, and a beautiful fall. It seemed very much like fall in Colorado, sunny blue skies and colorful trees. As I was unloading my moving truck some neighbors offered to help me schlep my belongings into my house. What a great place I had moved to, where strangers where willing to help "the new guy" haul stuff into his house without even knowing him!

The weather was indeed much like Colorado's, only a little colder. One day when the leaves were at peak color, a windstorm hit. Autumn was over. One moment the trees were full of yellow and orange leaves, the next moment they were bare and ready for winter. Cold weather moved in, and on Halloween the temperature was hovering around zero degrees. I began wondering if I would see any trick-or-treaters. If it had been this cold back in Colorado on Halloween I don't think I would have seen many ghouls on the streets. But Montana kids were tough, and many braved the cold in pursuit of the free candy available that night. The days continued to shrink in length, with sunrise starting later and later and the evening dusk arriving earlier and earlier.

I started work a few days after my arrival. I was settling into working a different system, one in which you work in the ER until a call drops. The advice I received early on by a veteran of the crew was to "not rock the boat or offer suggestions on how to change things until I had been there for a good long while and gotten used to how things were run." That seemed like good advice, although it was hard for me to keep my mouth quiet when I could see better ways to run things, like the way we did it back in the city. But I wanted to make friends and fit into the new system, so I wasn't about to rock the boat.

Running a call in Montana was not a whole lot different than running a call in Colorado. Things were a little more conservative as far as protocols were concerned, and I noticed that we were called "ambulance drivers" a lot – by the doctors, nurses and the general public. This didn't seem to bother the other people working on the ambulance so I didn't let it bother me.

But it was difficult because being called "ambulance driver" had bothered so many of my fellow EMS workers back in Colorado. We do so much more than just drive an ambulance.

I later came to find out that it had been only a few years since this town first started employing paramedics. As far as the attitude towards paramedicine was concerned, this place seemed about 10 years behind.

My working days in the ER were filled with doing 12-lead EKG's, starting IVs, checking vitals, running a call or two and taking patients admitted to the hospital to their rooms. Hanging out in the ER was pretty boring for me. I was accustomed to being in a base and doing my own thing until a call "dropped." It reminded me of being a bartender and spending my time wiping glasses to look busy.

Sometimes things at the ER were so slow it drove me crazy. The manager wanted us to look busy because he felt we had to justify our jobs. Back in Colorado, I had worked systems where you might only run a call or two a shift — or you could run up to 15 or more. It was all luck of the draw.

While working in the ER we still had plenty of time to talk and get to know our co-workers. I learned a lot about hunting and fishing because it was one of the main topics of conversation. I remember a conversation in which a nurse told the story of how her 15-year-old daughter had bagged her first bear. Life was different here. Young teenage girls hung out in malls where I came from, not out in the mountains looking for bears to kill. I started thinking

31

maybe it was time I went out shopping for a nice hunting rifle … and while I was at it, perhaps I should buy a pistol. Owning a gun seemed to be a part of living in Montana.

One of my fellow paramedics was a part-timer who was also the deputy sheriff. He had a wicked sense of humor and seemed to really know the people of the area. Another part-time paramedic was the person who kept the ambulances running. He did a fantastic job. It was different here: you couldn't just drive the rig to Denver to get it fixed, like I was used to.

We would take an ambulance to his shop for repair, and try to waste as much time as possible to stay out of the ER. There always seemed to be one or two locals hanging out, drinking coffee and just talking. Montana seemed like a place where people had time to be friendly. It seemed like the people who cared and worked hard in this town also felt strongly about helping people by taking care of the ambulances.

One of the first continuing education classes I took was about "Advanced Airways and Cricothyrotomies." I was given directions to one of the paramedic's ranches and told to show up by 6 p.m. Upon arriving, we all went to the barn where two sheep were being medicated by a local vet. Once the sheep had stopped moving but were still alive, we proceeded to practice "crics" on them. I have to admit I just couldn't do it. You can move the boy out of the city but you can't move the city out of the boy, as the saying goes.

It seemed to be a very effective training, making this procedure much more realistic than cutting into a piece of rubber covering a fake throat on some fake head. I'm still not sure how I feel about not wanting to cut into a live sheep trachea, and I'm sure a person would be different.

It wasn't until a few months into my Montana adventure that I realized it wasn't going to be quite the adventure I had hoped for.

Some of the differences I started to notice between the way I practice medicine and the way they did it in Montana started to get to me. For example, I was toned to a chest pain on a 55-year-old male. Upon arriving on scene, I found a slightly overweight male who was sweating profusely and described his chest pain as "8 out of 10" and radiating to his left arm. I loaded him up quick, got him into the back of the ambulance and got to work. I gave him aspirin and started an IV. After giving him nitroglycerin, I discovered he was allergic to morphine so I couldn't give him any of that. His EKG confirmed he was having a huge MI (myocardial infarction). I ended up giving him two more nitro and started a second IV en route to the ER. This is "good medicine," the way I was taught in Colorado.

Arriving at the ER less than five minutes later, I gave my report to the ER staff when my manager came in and started trying to take over. I was questioned by a nurse why I had chosen to start two lines. Frankly, I was starting to get pissed off. In my mind, I had just done a great job with this guy who was sick, while my manager got all hyped up and freaked out and a nurse questioned why I started two IVs.

Right about that time the patient went into V-tach and had a seizure and it was the biggest seizure I had ever seen. During the seizure one of his IVs got pulled out. Luckily I had started that second one. I looked over at the nurse, who didn't say anything. My boss was getting really wound up now.

I had to leave. It was time to restock the ambulance and get out of that crazy room. No "thank you's" or "atta-boys."

33

Later that day, I was questioned if the patient had been dropped because he had broken some bones. It was assumed that the ambulance crew must have dropped him because of his injuries. We had NOT and told them so. The doctors said later that it was possible he could have broken some bones during the seizure. It was a doozer of a seizure.

A week later I learned about a patient that another paramedic brought into the ER. The paramedic responded to a cardiac arrest, and when she dropped the patient off at the emergency room she didn't have the patient intubated, nor did she even attempt an IV. Basically, she did BLS (basic life support) stuff — CPR and bagged (rescue breathing for the patient with an ambubag) the patient. No attempt to intubate, push drugs — you know, paramedic stuff. The ER staff told her what a great job she did. It was beginning to dawn on me that we really were thought of as "ambulance drivers," and if we did more than that, it quickly became a bit suspect.

By the end of that winter, I was ready to leave.

My time in Montana had indeed been an adventure. I guess I missed the best time of year in Montana, which would be summer. I did meet a lot of great people whom I had befriended and come to admire.

I am impressed how the practice of paramedicine can be as different as night and day, yet the underlying theme of paramedics and EMTs who really do care about the job remains the same. They do the best job they can with the resources available.

Now living in Colorado again, I am grateful for the opportunity I had in Montana. I still think of the great people I met and worked with there and regret that it didn't work out a little better…

Or maybe I was meant to move back to Colorado and just enjoy the short adventure I had as an ambulance driver in Montana.

Chapter 6

Sometimes We Care Too Much

By Nick Hoskin

The Pearl Street Mall in Boulder, Colorado is a pedestrian mall that sits at the base of the foothills of the Rocky Mountains. It is a wonderful place to take the kids, wander around looking through store windows, watch people, and grab a bite to eat.

It is the classic, late-summer Boulder day on the mall, crowded with people and sidewalk sales — not too hot and not too cold. I am walking on the West End of the mall with my 2-year-old little girl holding my hand and my 5-year-old son a few feet ahead. I see a 20-something male sitting on a public bench fast asleep, who appears to be a transient. I am unconcerned because this often happens on the Pearl Street Mall, and I wasn't working that day. Plus, I had my kids with me, so I wasn't about to go up and wake this guy to see if he was OK.

I met up with my wife, who had gone ahead to do some shopping without the kids. We all spend about 10 minutes together looking at some of the sales outside on the sidewalk. On our way back to the car I see a police officer trying to wake up the 20-something transient male. The officer looks like he could use a little help, so I go over and tell him who I am and ask if he needs assistance. He states that he has called for fire and ambulance non-emergent, and that they are on there way.

I give the young man a painful sternal rub, but he doesn't budge. He is breathing at a rate of about eight times a minute, so I am not too worried about his airway. My wife and kids are hanging out nearby, as my wife explains to my son that this is what Daddy does for work. Prying open the patient's eyelids, I see his pupils are pinpoint, which is a positive sign for narcotic use. Again, this is not an uncommon occurrence in Boulder, and I knew that after the patient received some Narcan, which immediately reverses the effects of narcotics, he would wake up and live to see another day.

Fire shows up, and I tell them what I know so far. They pick him up and place him on the ground. I suggest that they put a nasal pharyngeal airway (NPA) in his nose. They size up the proper NPA to use, lube it up with K-Y Jelly, and slide it in. The patient doesn't move, he is pretty far down. They put a non-rebreather on him and keep him oxygenated. After checks of his blood pressure and pulse, the ambulance shows up. Two of my co-workers arrive, both of whom I like and trust. Mark is a long-time medic who received his training down in Knoxville, Tenn. He moved to Colorado a few years prior because he needed a change in his environment. His partner, Molly, is a seasoned EMT.

As Mark gets out of the ambulance and sees me, a smile crosses his face. He looks at the patient and says they had heard that the patient had been intubated and that they were questioning if they heard that right over the radio. It turns out that the police officer had confused his medical terminology and thought that when fire inserted an NPA that meant he was intubated.

Mark and Molly load the patient into the back of the ambulance. I hang out as they start an IV. Mark pulls out the Narcan. I see him push just a little and then I see him get real close to the patient's ear and whisper something to him.

I ask if they need any more help. "No thanks, Nick, you've been more than enough help already," Mark says with a small smile on his face, as if to say, "Let the sleeping heroin addict sleep."

At work the next day I ask Mark what he whispered to the patient. He sighs a little and proceeds to tell me a story of why he left Tennessee.

"Nick, I grew up on the rough side of Knoxville and became a paramedic because I wanted to help people. I had spent my youth fighting and partying, and I had seen quite a few of my friends die from OD'ing on heroin. I love being a paramedic and feel like I have done a lot of good helping people. But one thing I don't have any tolerance for is people doing heroin. So, whenever I run on somebody like I did yesterday, I start a line, give them a little Narcan to wake them up just enough to hear me. I get down real close to their ear so I know they can hear me. I asked him, 'How would your grandma feel going to your funeral because you died doing heroin? How can you be such a selfish prick to do this?'" he said.

Mark looks kind of sad as he continues. "I've buried three of my friends who took that shit. It's just a waste."

"That sucks, Mark. I'm sorry" I reply.

He looks at me and gets this big shit-eating grin on his face and says, "Thanks, man, but the best part is that after I saw a couple of tears roll out of that dude's eye yesterday, and I knew he got my message, I slammed the rest of the Narcan into him to take him off his high fast and make him remember this day. Stupid fucker." He laughed.

It didn't take me long to realize how much Mark cares

about this. I've never had a friend die from heroin. I can see a part of me wanting to judge Mark for being mean and uncaring to that guy, but I think Mark might have given that guy the best care in the world. I bet that kid's grandma would thank Mark if she knew what he did for her grandson.

Chapter 7

First Day

By Steve Smith

This is my first shift on an ALS (advance life support) ambulance. Yesterday I was on a BLS (basic life support) transport ambulance. I've been promoted for one day because we are short on staff and I volunteered for the shift. After finding out that management accepted my offer, I am feeling pretty nervous. I haven't even driven "emergent" yet.

I get stuck working with this crusty old medic, who started working in this county when I was 7 years old.

We start our shift at 5:30 a.m. and Nick, the crusty old medic, starts talking about his philosophy of paramedicine. He tells me a few things about what he expects from me. Then he goes off on tangents about how he believes an ambulance company should work, how all privates are pretty much the same, and how EMTs need to mold to the medic. He's not surprised to be working with a green EMT who has had no training. This is what private ambulances do — they don't pay people well enough to make them stick around and then they are short people and try to fill the seat with somebody who has a heartbeat. He says the company should figure out how to hold onto employees instead of just putting a warm body in the seat. Then he grabs a ratty old pillow, curls it up in a ball, stuffs that pillow into the door jam, closes his eyes and goes to sleep. I put my head back and close my eyes, hoping to get some sleep myself. *What have I gotten myself into?*

The tone goes off. My heart starts beating way too fast as adrenaline pumps through my veins. The fire department outside our area is toned to a car accident. Nick doesn't even stir. Forty-five minutes later, listening to Nick snore finally comes to an end when he wakes up and pronounces it time for breakfast. In between bites of his bagel and sips of coffee, he imparts more of his philosophy. Some of it makes sense and actually helps me feel a little more at ease, such as, "Don't worry too much because I am the one who is in charge. I am responsible for everything, not you. I won't let you screw up too much because then it would be my ass."

Nick also tells me that if he deems it OK, he will let me have the patient.

Nick is the one driving emergent on the first call. The lights and sirens are going. He is chattering away about watching for other cars, weaving in and out of traffic, calling the cars that stop in the middle of the road "ding-dongs" — all the while trying to teach me how to drive emergent.

I am navigating, and I get us lost because I direct us down the wrong road. I find where we were supposed to go, and we finally got to the call. It is called in as a 71-year-old female who is feeling weak. Fire is already on scene, and I am feeling a little overwhelmed, lost and unsure of what to do. Nick is standing back listening to what fire says. He finally goes up to the patient and starts talking with her. He tells me to get the pram, which I do. I come back trying to catch up with what is going on, in case I am given this patient on the way to the hospital.

Nick ends up attending on this call. He talks about patients being "sick" or "not sick." I think this guy is sick! But the patient doesn't seem very sick to me, and I wonder why I am not given this call. I ask Nick, and he says it is because he doesn't trust me yet. *Okay, that's fair, I guess... Man, this is going be a long day.*

Before I volunteered for this shift, I knew I was going to be getting on an ALS ambulance. My plan was that as soon as I started on ALS, I would start to eat healthier and stop chewing. While I am not officially training on an ALS ambulance today, I am working on one, if even for a day. So this is my first day of not chewing, and I explain it to Nick. He asks me *why*. I explain, "Because I don't like the habit, and I don't want to get cancer."

"You'll need a bigger *why* than that," he laughed. "Plus, you are about to be under a lot of stress, and you want to give up chewing now?" What a jerk. I am ready to do this.

On our next call, I drive emergent and I almost stack up our ambulance and feel ragged. I pull into a gas station, buy a can of chew and stick in a pinch. It tastes good. *What a jerk, making me chew again.* However, it does calm my nerves. Maybe he is right. If some guy saying that this is not the time to stop is all it took for me to chew, perhaps his idea of having a big enough *why* makes a little more sense. Whatever. I still think he is a jerk.

We cancel on some older guy who has low blood sugar. We head to a transfer (taking a patient from one facility to another), just like I do on the BLS transfer van, and I get to attend. Then right after that we go to the ARC (alcohol recovery center) on a guy who is not feeling well. This guy isn't sick, but we take him to the hospital. Nick lets me attend. "What are you going to do?" Nick asks.

"I guess I'll put him on some oxygen and start a line," I reply.

"Why don't you *do* that! But you shouldn't guess. Do it! How would you like some paramedic to *guess* what drug he might push into your Mom if she was sick," Nick says as he shuts the doors. What a prick.

I get all the stuff ready. The hospital is close, so I hurry. I put a tourniquet on the patient's arm and look for a vein. We are bouncing down the road, and I wait for a smooth place. It feels like Nick is intentionally hitting every hole and bump he can. I go to stick the needle in, and we hit a bump. I pull back. I can see a drop of blood start to pool. I stick the needle in right above the drop of blood and level out the IV, just like I learned in class. Blood fills up the flash chamber. I'm in. I attach the vacutainer hub and draw blood. I hook up the NS (normal saline) and put it to TKO (to keep open). I have successfully gotten in my first IV in the back of a bumpy, moving ambulance, shaking hands and all. We drop our patient off at the hospital, and I tell the nurse his story. This feels like the first real call I attended on. I feel pretty good.

We go park in the middle of town because we are the only ambulance in service. A tone drops for a party with a head injury at the soccer fields. I'm driving emergent for the second time. The butterflies in my stomach seem to be flying faster than I am driving. I back up the ambulance close to the field and find out the patient was playing rugby, not soccer. We start pulling spinal immobilization equipment out of the back of the rig when a guy runs up, tells us to hurry, he thinks the patient is having a heart attack. We throw the backboard and c-collar back in the ambulance and grab the monitor. On the sideline, there is an older guy lying down on the grass. Nick seems to switch gears, transforming from some crusty old fart who doesn't give a shit about anything to the all-business paramedic who is totally in control.

"Hi, what's your name?" Nick asks.

"Tim", the patient says.

"What seems to be going on today?"

Tim proceeds to tell Nick that his chest is hurting, and no, it doesn't get worse when you push on it or when I take a deep breath. It's about an 8 on the scale of 0-to-10, 10 being the worst. Tim is all sweaty and looks pretty sick.

Nick explains that he is putting on some oxygen. He messes around with the oxygen tank and then puts it down, without putting oxygen on and without a word. He just grabs the life pack and puts on the heart monitor. Fire shows up, and Nick tells them to get the patient on oxygen. I wonder why he didn't do it himself. He must think it is an EMT job or something. I'm trying to get the blood pressure. I can't hear one. I contemplate making one up, but I remember Nick saying earlier not to make stuff up and to trust myself with blood pressures and stuff like that.

Nick cups his hands around the monitor so he can see it in the bright sunlight. All of a sudden Nick commands, "Get him loaded up. Expedite!" He then tells me to run ahead and spike a bag of saline. I get to the ambulance, pull out a bag of saline and start to get it ready. Nick shows up, kicks me out and tells me to get up front. I'm getting the impression that this guy is really sick.

I'm told to drive emergent to the hospital, "nice and easy." Up front with me is the patient's wife. She is asking me questions about her husband, and I'm not sure how to answer them. I miss the turn to the hospital and have to go around the block. I've made this turn a hundred times on transfers before. God, how did I become such an idiot?

We drop the patient off, and Nick tells me he was having "the big one." Tim was having a massive MI (myocardial infarction or heart attack). He was sick. Tim ended up having quadruple bypass surgery.

Nick then proceeds to tell me that the reason he didn't put oxygen on the guy when we first got there is because the portable oxygen tank was empty.

"It is your responsibility to keep on top of that stuff," Nick chastised, "Plus there wasn't a nasal cannula in the bag. We're lucky AND the patient is lucky that fire showed up with their oxygen."

I pull the can of chew out of my pocket and put in a big ole dip. Nick was right about the stress. Mainly all I was doing was driving and I screwed that up, not to mention the oxygen. I thought, *"Man, I suck, this stuff is stressful. It really can be about life and death."*

That is the last call of our shift. We head back to base. Nick starts spouting more of his philosophy. And then surprises me with, "Steve, you did good today."

In rebuttal, "I missed the turn and had to drive around the block … and then the oxygen thing." I am feeling pretty upset. At least I didn't give up chewing, because I needed that today.

Nick continues, "Yeah, you missed a turn, but you got us to the ER eventually. I'll also bet in the future you check your oxygen more often. Mistakes are our best teachers. We learn best from screwing up. The secret is to not beat yourself up too much. Learn from your mistakes, and move on. It is called 'practicing medicine' for a reason. We are practicing all the time. No one is perfect. If others say they don't screw up, they are either liars, or they are full of shit.

"You did well today, Steve. I think you will do great in the field. Remember it takes about a year to feel comfortable. It was fun working with you."

Then he says something about being a hero and saving a life. Then he laughs this cynical little laugh like he knows he was full of shit.

That was it. He does his end-of-shift stuff and goes home. I am still buzzing from the day. I started an IV in the back of a moving ambulance, drove emergent, saw a guy having a big MI, and made it through my first ALS shift. It was great. I screwed up a couple of times, but it was still great. I think I am going to love this work. In the end, I realize that Nick is OK. He is a crusty, old fart, but I think he really does care. He taught me a thing or two that will help me in the field, and I guess it could have been a lot worse.

Chapter 8

On The Job

By Floyd Salazar

I don't remember my first call. I don't remember the first time I went into a burning building. I don't remember the first time I saw a dead body or the first time I told someone that their somebody had died, that we'd done all we could but that someone died. One would think I'd remember my excitement, dread and/or fear surrounding these firsts, which were assuredly separate events, but I have no recollection of the details.

I do remember my very first shift on the line. I left my bunker pants at the house when we went on a medical call. I remember a weekend morning early in my career when I put too much vanilla extract in the pancake batter and the resulting cakes had the consistency and moisture content of cinder blocks. I remember the first time I bought ice cream for my crew because some TV videographer got me on tape and the segment aired on a local TV news broadcast — it was at a fire where a kid got burned to death when he was playing with a lighter. I remember the fire very well, but don't have particularly strong memories of the kid.

I'm a firefighter/paramedic. I used to think that those jobs went together as naturally as chocolate and peanut butter: two good things that go good together. But often, when people ask me what I do, after hearing my reply they say, "Well which one are you?"

47

"I'm both."

They look at me perplexed, as if I just gave them an impassioned diatribe on the income tax system of southern Romania. I understand, though. For folks not in the business, they don't understand why a fire engine comes screaming up the street when they called for an ambulance. They don't understand that the fire department's people and equipment is strategically placed to reach any address is very short order, sometimes as quickly as two to four minutes but never more than eight minutes. In the city where I work (and this is true in most cities) there are more fire engines than ambulances, so it takes longer for the ambulance to get to the call. In an effort to get help to the call faster, at least one of the four people on the fire engine is a paramedic.

Rather than explaining all that, I usually tell people I herd cats.

When I'm talking with folks who are in the business, the question is, "Where do you work?"

When I say I work for the BLANK fire department, the conversation takes a different turn.

If a private or government or hospital-subsidized EMS agency (no firefighters here, thanks very much) employs the person I'm speaking with, I'm assessed with quiet skepticism. It's very logical and not intended or taken rudely. After all, my fire department does not have any ambulances. So what kind of paramedic can I be if I've never worked on an ambulance? There is a big rift between us — the folks who work fire and do EMS and the folks who work only EMS.

As a paramedic in a fire department, I make more and do

less work than my private sector counterparts. I'm a member of a union that negotiates for my pay and benefits. The fire department I belong to has a mandatory retirement plan, so I'm forced to save money, which puts me and my compatriots in a better financial position that most of the American working class. The hierarchy of the fire department allows for a career ladder that employees can progress through. Even many large, private-sector EMS agencies have only a handful of supervisor positions. My department has over 50 such positions. When I come to work I get to live in a firehouse, whereas they often spend their entire shift in their ambulance.

On the flip side, as a firefighter/paramedic the folks from my own department regard me and those like me with a kind of pathetic curiosity. Back in the 1970's, paramedics were regarded with the special kind of loathing usually reserved for folks that answer their cell phones in the theater. Today most firefighters feel sorry for us. They proclaim to anyone who'll listen, "Why the hell would anyone want to be a paramedic?" They spit out the word "paramedic" like it's a mouthful of sour milk. We have more bosses than they do. We have to do more training and more paperwork. We carry all the legal responsibility for the EMS calls, which incidentally makes up 70 percent of our total workload. But the fire department is a big extended family and we never miss an opportunity to convey support to one another. Paramedics in my outfit are commonly referred to as "pecker checkers" or "dick smiths," though being called a "gutter nurse" is a mark of high praise.

Paramedics tell me I can't be a really good paramedic. Firefighters tell me I can't be a really good firefighter.

Why would anyone be a firefighter/paramedic? It's a good question, one for which I have a difficult time articulating an answer.

In 1991 my fire department had 36 paramedics staffing six rigs that answered just under 12,000 calls. In 2007 we have 43 paramedics staffing 15 rigs that answered almost 20,000 calls. Apparently I'm not the only one who has a hard time answering the question. Since we can't get enough guys to volunteer to become paramedics, we now mandate paramedic training as a condition of employment. It hasn't been a popular decision.

Shit happens and people call the fire department, no matter what kind of emergency it is. When they call they expect paramedics, never mind that only one or two of the people there is in fact a paramedic. Nationwide, there are fewer fires and more medical emergencies. Fire departments are staffed up to fight fires, but the gap in demand for emergency medical services is filled by specialist paramedics. As our population ages and healthcare costs continue to skyrocket, 911 is the number for any medical complaint. We are called upon daily to assist people who do not really require emergency care. Even those that can afford healthcare will call 911 because they think if they go to the hospital in an ambulance they won't have to sit in the waiting room for hours on end.

Rather than snatching our patients from the jaws of crippling tragedy, we are more often called to make basic decisions for people. Do I need to see a doctor? If so, do I have to see the emergency room doctor, or can I make an appointment with my primary care physician? If I do need to see an emergency room doctor, do I need a ride in an ambulance or can my wife drive me? The reality is that we are the people you call when you don't have anyone else to call.

I remember a call where a little old lady needed us to turn off her television. She had misplaced the remote so she just started pushing buttons on the set. The lettering marking the buttons was too small for her to read. She'd inadvertently turned the volume up so loud, I thought the *Rolling Stones* were doing a sound check in her living room.

People call when their fillings fall out. They call when they are so drunk they can't take care of themselves. They call because the water pipes have frozen, thawed and busted and they need help dealing with the landlord who won't return their phone calls. They call from their nursing home beds because "they won't bring me my damn cookies." They call because they are afraid and want someone to tell them it'll be OK. They call because they are lonely.

A lot of guys will bitch about these "garbage runs" because it wasn't what they signed on for. We are the fire department. We are here to save lives. We aren't supposed to put Band-Aids on kids with boo-boos on their knees. We aren't supposed to babysit drunks trying to dry up. We aren't supposed to run on the same junkie who has overdosed three times in the same day. We aren't supposed to run lights and sirens to some idiot who found an empty can of spray paint in the gutter and wants to know if it's safe to pick up and throw in the trash.

Well I got news for you: That is exactly our job. We help people who cannot help themselves. That is who we are, and that is our mission. If you think being a firefighter would be a pretty cool gig but can't fathom being pooped on or touching sick people, this is not the gig for you. We have lots of folks that work fire and do EMS. We need people that want to work fire and EMS.

EMS is a tough thing to wrap one's mind around because it's a futile pursuit.

Of course everybody wants to save a life. Not because you want heroic notoriety but you crave the respect of your peers. You want to be seen as a guy your peers can count on to do your share.

But such opportunities are misleading or very rare. In the instances where people are trapped in burning buildings, it is easy to see the direct relationship between firefighters' actions and saved lives. The engine company puts out the fire while the truck company rescues the family from the balcony. The battle is clear cut, cleanly fought, and the results are immediate. You can see them, folks that were in danger of burning to death just minutes ago, standing on the street holding one another crying, and there is no doubt in your mind they all would've died if the firefighters hadn't saved them.

But most of the time, we are trying to save people from the cheeseburgers and beers they've been ingesting for the last 40 years. We are trying to save a lady from the hundreds of thousands of cigarettes she's smoked over a lifetime. We are trying to deny the asthma suffocating a man long enough to get him to a team of doctors that might be able to save him. We are trying to save a child born with ailments so severe that the child's parents have had to learn to suction blocked airways or administer life-preserving medicines before we even arrive. We are trying to free someone from a pile of twisted metal that was a car.

The reality is that most of these battles are lost long before they have begun. After all, the defining element of human existence is our mortality. People die. Every day, people die.

And yet we are still out there. It has been said that firefighters are soldiers in a war that never ends. It is also a war that can never be won, a fire that can never be extinguished.

Shift after shift. Sleepless night after sleepless night. As guys get seniority, they transfer to slower houses and encourage the younger guys to do the same. It's a job where the pay is the same whether you get up six times after midnight or you sleep like a baby, if such a thing is possible in a firehouse.

And when you are called to work at a real emergency, you find yourself participating in the most horrendous events. You work trying to sustain the life of a young woman who was going to get married the next month. You know this because her bridal gown is hanging in what used to be her car and her leftover invitations are scattered all over the road. You work on a small child burned so badly that the grime covering your gloves is not blood but human fat that seeped from the open cracks in the charred flesh. You watch a young girl cry while her mother, who was cooking meth in the same kitchen she fed her daughter from, is being carted off to jail. You find yourself in these moments, and you ask yourself, "What the hell am I doing here?"

A close friend of mine told me every night at work as he is trying to go to sleep, he experiences overwhelming moments of terror as he agonizes over if his daughter is all right. "If I was at home," he said, "I'd just walk down the hall and peek in her room. Can't do that from the firehouse. So I just lie there and shake for a while. At least until we get a call."

There is no other organization in the world that can promise what we deliver every day at any hour.

Churches lock their doors. Doctors do not make house calls, and the after-hours clinics close at around 11 p.m. Therapists go on vacation. Insurance companies deny claims. You might be able to get it made your way at Burger King, but don't try that at McDonald's. If you call the cops, it may be hours before they show up. But when people call the fire department, the fire department will come. No questions asked. It is easy to forget that unspoken unconditional commitment and the power that commitment entails.

When I think of it, that is what compelled me to be a firefighter/paramedic. Not because I wanted to be a hero. Not because the work schedule is great. Not because the union sticker on my car window gets me out of the occasional speeding ticket.

These are the guys that don't give up. They take gleeful joy in tormenting one another but then they come back to the firehouse after a tough run and sit on the bumper and cry for strangers. These are the guys that will get into screaming matches over the TV remote or almost come to blows over a presidential candidate, but when the tones ring down they are ready to place their lives in each other's hands.

Fire is immortal and people are not. Even in the face of that inevitable existential truth, these are the guys that are never afraid to stand up and take a swing and then take a fall, only to pick themselves up and wait for, hope for, another chance to face the gods again, even if it means losing again.

Joss Whedon said, "If nothing that we do matters, then the only thing that matters is what we do." I have yet to hear a better explanation of why I'm a firefighter/paramedic.

Chapter 9

Scrabble

By Mollie McGirk

It started out a normal day for me. I wake up late, throw on my uniform, hopefully remembering to put on deodorant and head into work only to experience a little road rage as I blame everyone else in the world for my being late to work. I screech around the corner as I see my partner screeching around the other corner, both of us with two minutes to clock in and get on the streets. The team leader just shakes his head as we burst through the doors with shirts untucked, boots unzipped, grinning as we high five each other. "Juuust made it!"

We put ourselves in service. We have a little ritual. I ask my partner, "What do you want to do today?" To which he usually responds, "Play Scrabble!" But today he says, "Let's run something good today!" I curse him for jinxing us. I am sure that we will now be plagued with lame transfers all day long.

We get posted in one of the slowest parts of the county and in my mind I hear children laughing and bells sounding, because I'm going to get a nap! Oh, how I love to sleep.

As we pull into town, he asks for coffee. We pull up to the coffee shop and a tone drops, as it never fails to do, for a fallen party across the street. I can literally see the apartment complex from where we are sitting.

55

"A fall, how exciting," I say in my most sarcastic voice. We are so close we don't even turn the lights or siren on because it would be more of a hassle. We consider canceling the fire department's response because they are coming from so far away, but decide against it. We pull around the corner and I see what an old partner of mine used to refer to as the obligatory waver — the person that makes the silliest hand gestures waving down the ambulance as we pull up — standing at the door of a third level apartment.

I laugh to myself as I think of the movie "Bringing out the Dead" when John Goodman says, "Why is it always the third floor?"

I look at my partner and say, "Wow, she's frantic!" Something is odd. We get out of the ambulance and hear her say, "HURRY, HURRY!!"

"WE'RE COMING, GOD!!" I am screaming in my mind. I grab a backboard, and my partner grabs the kit and monitor. We start to head up the stairs with him in the lead. He is a little ways ahead of me because I am trying to carry the oxygen and backboard and I keep dropping things. Out of nowhere I see my partner (keep in mind he's been called a lot of things, never though has he been called tiny) barreling down the stairs at me throwing the med kit in the grass, and all I hear is, "She shot herself in the fucking head!" Which would explain the fall. It's hard to stand when you do that, or so I hear.

HEEELLLP!!! I think as we run for shelter behind the ambulance. *Wait, we are the help!* Still alone on scene, my partner calls PD (police department) in emergent because it sounds like there are more people in the apartment, and we are unsure who the shooter was. PD arrives and they start running up the stairs. PD checks out the scene and says it is code four, it is safe for us to come in. We find a woman, our patient, seated on her balcony bleeding from the head. My partner who has been a paramedic for six or so months (but an EMT for several years prior to that) has not yet gotten a tube (intubation) outside of paramedic school. He is having trouble intubating the patient, and the other treatments we are trying to get done are not going well either.

This woman has what looks like an abdominal wound with her intestines leaking out. It turns out to be a pool of clotted blood that leaked from the hole in her head onto her abdomen. This only adds to the confusion. We are unable to intubate her on scene, so my partner says to move her to the ambulance. I told the firefighters to spike blood pumps in the ambulance. Then I realized how dumb that was, so I spiked blood pumps in the apartment because we were going to start an IV on scene. At the end of this call there were probably four or five blood pumps spiked. We left a mess of bloody endotracheal tubes and other garbage on the floor, so I look at the FD guys and ask if they'll take the patient down the stairs. Amidst all of the stress, we forget to put a blanket over the patient's now exposed chest. Don't get me wrong, maintaining a patient's dignity is important, but it just slipped our minds.

She is taken down the stairs exposed from waist up. My partner gets the patient intubated en route to the hospital. We finally deliver this patient to the hospital, yet this patient is still successful in her wanting to die despite our paramount attempts to save her life. This was a stressful call to say the least. Scene safety is something that I had begun to take for granted, and that is not something I am proud of. It can be easy to get lulled into a false sense of security. We were both stressed out from that call and ready to go home.

As we pull back into the station that evening, I hear my

57

shift supervisor on the phone obviously handling a complaint. A woman called to complain about our call. How dare we let breasts be exposed to the public. So much for a thank-you. I joked with my partner to get his priorities straight.

As we headed out the door on our way home, I ask, "What do you want to do tomorrow?"

To which he replies, "Play Scrabble".

Chapter 10

I'm a good girl

T.J. Avischious

Just over three years ago, I was doing my emergency room (ER) rotation for EMT school. I was 19 years old, and I admit, a little wet around the ears. I was assigned to a nurse, Amy, who had been around for quite a while. It was a night shift and things were pretty slow. A couple of minor cases had come in — nausea/vomiting, lacerations that needed to be sutured, general stuff. These types of cases were routine for me because I had been a volunteer for the past nine months at a local fire department, where I'd seen some cool stuff.

It was still early in my shift when a mom came in with her 5-year-old daughter on one hand and a 3-month-old in her other arm. The mom had a good hold on her daughter's arm and was dragging her into the triage room. She was a single mom in her early 30s and she looked a little tired around the eyes, kind of worn-down — the kind of mom who looked like she really didn't know how to deal with the stress of parenting. They came to the ER because the mom's hand was red and swollen, and it wasn't getting any better.

This was a small enough hospital where the nurse I was following was doing triage out front and taking care of patients in the back. Amy had me checking the patient's blood pressure and pulse while she started asking questions.

"Are you allergic to anything, medications or food?" Amy asked.

"No," Mom answered.

"Did you eat anything out of the ordinary or have you been in contact with anything that might have caused this?" Amy asked.

"No, not a thing." was Mom's reply.

"What were you doing when this started?" was Amy's next question.

"Well, we, the kids and I, were sitting down to dinner when this started. We were eating dinner and I asked Lisa — this is Lisa here, she's 5 — I asked her to spell 'cat.' Lisa kept spelling it 'K-A-T.' I told her so many times how to spell it and she couldn't do it, so I hit her with my hand."

"How many times did you hit her with your hand? 10?" Amy asked.

"Oh, it was way more than that," Mom stated, matter-of-factly.

"20, 30, 40?" Amy followed up.

"I don't even know, it was so many times....I don't know....maybe 50...yeah, I'd say closer to 50," she replied.

Amy wanted to clarify, "You hit your 5-year-old daughter, Lisa, 50 times with your hand?"

"Yeah, I'd say 50. Then my hand started hurting so bad I

had to use a belt," she said, as if this was a normal thing for a mom to do.

"You hit your daughter with a belt after your hand started hurting, and you did this because your daughter couldn't spell the word cat, is this correct?" Amy said.

"Yeah." said mom, without much regret or concern in her voice.

My brain, all my senses were screaming at me to hit this woman, to protect this little girl. I had to concentrate and calm down, force my fists to uncurl and relax. I didn't understand how Amy, a nurse who is supposed to care about people, could be so calm and relaxed. I wanted to kill this lady.

"OK ma'am, let's go back to Room 3 so we can take a look at your hand and see what we can do," Amy said in the sweetest of voices.

The five of us walked back to Room 3. Amy asked the mom to sit on the bed and to relax. Amy then asked me to sit on a stool at a desk that had a good view of Room 3. "Don't take your eyes off of that woman, and if she touches her daughter in any way, you come and get me, I'll be right back," Amy told me forcibly.

Maybe Amy wasn't as calm and cool as she had appeared; maybe she was as pissed off as me.

Mom was in the room pacing. She would go to one side and stare at me and then to the other side of the room and stare at her older daughter. During this time, Amy and the other nurses where talking with the doctor to figure out what to do. The police were called, along with social services.

The police officer who arrived joined Amy and the doctor. Mom started to look a little more agitated and paced a little faster. I went into the room with two other nurses and we had mom step out of the room without her little girls. The nurses took mom around the corner, and the police officer put our patient into handcuffs.

One of the other nurses started to take care of the 3-month-old. Amy and I started to take care of Lisa. We wanted to check Lisa over for any injury and started to get her undressed. We were taking her out of her pants and she cringed, pulling back a bit as if it hurt. The upper backsides of her legs were covered in scarlet, vicious-looking welts. Her buttocks were all red and swollen. She could barely stand. We had to weigh her and she couldn't stand on the scale, she had to sit down. There may have been some old bruising, but it was hard to tell.

"Where is my Mommy?" Lisa asked.

"She had to go somewhere. TJ here is going to take care of you for a while," Amy answered.

My heart was breaking. How could anyone hit a child like Lisa?

After the doctor thoroughly checked over Lisa and her sister, I spent the rest of the evening hanging out with Lisa. We talked some, I found a coloring book and crayons, and we found some snacks and apple juice.

I asked Lisa what she wanted to do when she grew up.

"I want to be a ballerina," she answered. Then, "Why does my mom hit me? I'm a good girl."

That was it. Any resolve I had in not crying burst. Tears began streaming down my face. "I don't know why your mom hits you, but you are a beautiful young girl, and you don't deserve to be hit in any way," I replied.

She moved onto being a ballerina again and drank some apple juice. It was getting late and the evening's events had taken their toll on Lisa and she fell asleep. She looked like a little angel sleeping in that hospital bed.

The social worker showed up and filled out a bunch of paperwork. Lisa slept like a baby. Lisa's grandparents showed up and took the two little girls home.

It was close to 3 a.m. and time for me to go home. I felt raw and still angry at Lisa's mom. How could somebody do this? As I was walking out the door, the exhaustion hit me. I had been on an emotional roller coaster for hours, going from complete rage to complete sorrow. I felt too tired to sleep, too exhausted to move.

Training to be a new EMT, I thought the job was about saving lives, doing CPR, making a difference. Tonight I had a different view on being an EMT. EMTs do make a difference, just in a much different way than I realized.

Chapter 11

A Day In The Life

By Lana Bond

Bored, bored, bored … Yup, yup, yup. Bored.

You know it's a slow day when you realize you've been watching the little guy get run down by the gorilla in the little cartoon game at the top of your MySpace page for the last minute and a half and thought it was interesting.

My partner and I sat in our ambulance for an hour this morning and speculated on the interest level of various calls: guy shoots himself in the head: 3; evisceration: 5; evisceration by samurai sword: 7; amputation: 2; hiker struck by lightening: 9; parachuter tangled in electrical lines: 10.

And so on.

Sick, yes, but oh so entertaining.

We're listening to overrated Dave Matthews and waiting to go home. We've been doing this for five hours. Well, we've been doing the first part for five hours. We've been doing the second part for 12 hours.

It's beautiful and quiet outside today, sunny, the stillness broken by the diesel hum of our ambulance engine.

There is a young man working on his red jeep in the parking lot in front of us. He has his pants cuffs rolled until they are flood tide. He has his rusty baseball cap on backward (crookedly). He has a massive case of plumber butt.

It's air-conditioning cold in this ambulance. My partner is drumming on his computer in time to the music and driving me crazy

What's *this?!?* A *call???* *OH JOY!!!* An MVA (car crash)! Lights! Sirens! Action! Wail. Screech. UTL (unable to locate). Of course (of curse). U-turn. Back to post. Sigh.

What a pretty day it is outside. My bum has gone to sleep from boredom. The sun is shining (but only one side of it, the right side — my bum, not the sun.) The air is crisp but not frigid. It's too warm for my poofy jacket but too cold to go without. I could put on my sweater, but it's scratchy and too big. Like many things in life, it almost but just doesn't quite fit. My finger joints ache. Shoes unzipped. Mom's the size of the dot at the end of this sentence. Cold coffee. Weather great until my day off ...

Last Wednesday I worked with the guy who may be one of the biggest reasons I decided to get into EMS. My first proctor. He was the paramedic on my very first "third ride" (when a student rides along in an ambulance for a shift) for my EMT class. Great storyteller. (Whenever he walked into the room and said, "So the other day ... " you know to just sit back and enjoy the tale.) Which is why I became interested in working on an ambulance. All the fascinating stories! What I didn't realize at the time is that 15 years of EMS stories action-packed into one 12-hour shift makes the job seem much more exciting than it usually is. "Catching butterflies" ("Hold it *gently...* it's *delicate!*") for acid trippers to keep them still. Dodging projectile-vomited bloody emesis. Army guys, prostitutes and STD's.

I suppose I have a few stories too.

I once had a man pray to me (that's right — *to* me.) I held his Bible like a blessing as I realized that he thought I was "enlightened."

I once made a crazy man who was convinced demons were after him, who attacked the staff at the hospital, who was under arrest for assault, cry. He was so concerned for my safety out there on those dangerous streets.

I once convinced a woman that it didn't matter if the government had bugged her house and job with cameras and microphones and spies because she wasn't doing anything wrong. *Was she??*

I once had a patient fall in love with me. ("Why do you drink so much?" "Because I love you TOO much! How come you won't kiss me?" "Because, Sir, grown women don't like men who pee their pants. ")

I once watched a little girl on her bike get hit by a car. She was fine.

One night (the same night) a man blew his brains out in the basement while his wife was vacuuming upstairs. He had blue eyes. He had the biggest head I have ever seen. He had brains sticking out of his huge head just above his left ear. He bled and bled and bled. He left a trail of life in a puddle under his chair and in a drip-drizzle up the stairs and out the garage and into our ambulance and in a coagulated mass under the sheet of our pram and into the shoe of the fire-medic who was trying to intubate him. He died.

His wife had dark, curly hair. She heard a bang. She turned off the vacuum. She listened. She heard the vents in the house. She turned the vacuum back on. She finished the upstairs. She went downstairs. She cried.

One time I went to a nursing home and saw a woman in a wheelchair. "I need to pay my bill," she tugged at my sleeve, her voice distressed, and her lined face tragic with eternal stress. "I *need* to pay my bill." I picked up and read the note cards tied to the arm of her chair. "I have Alzheimer's. I always believe that I have a bill that needs to be paid. Tell me that my family has paid for everything." I tell her. Her face settles into peace. She leans back. I walk away. I walk by again. It's been five minutes. She tugs at my sleeve. "I need to pay my *bill!*" There are tears in her eyes. I read the cards to her again. She settles back. She pulls her sweater around her shoulders. She shivers. Five minutes. She tugs at someone else's sleeve. I go home. I cry.

An old, old man in a nursing home plays the piano and sings. It is so beautiful.

One time a man went into cardiac arrest at Urgent Care. We shocked him and brought him back. By the time we got him to the hospital (which is across the street), he was trying to pull his tube. He had a tattoo on his arm that said "lucky."

One time we saved a life.

But today we sit. We sit. We wait. We wait. We wait. Add coffee. Add blogs. Add moving posts. Ad nauseum. Ad *tedium*. We clack at our computers. *Sigh*. We pick at each other. We annoy each other. We laugh at each other. We sit. We wait.

Sigh.

A day in the life.

Chapter 12

Snake Bite

By Nick Hoskin

It was early summer and the day had been quiet. We maybe had one call earlier, but we were working in a sleepy little bedroom community that didn't have a lot of action. Around 5 p.m. my partner Billy and I were toned to a snake bite. While I was driving, I was joking about how some kid must have been bitten by a garden snake and was freaking out. Sure, there are rattlesnakes in Colorado, but not in the town where we were working. The ambulance unit and fire units were in route and an update was being given.

"Paramedic 2 and Fire you are responding to a 51-year-old female who has her hand caught in a python's mouth."

"Wow, I guess this isn't a garden snake" I said and laughed.

I looked over at my partner to see if he was also laughing. He wasn't. He had a pretty serious expression on his face. I thought nothing of this as Billy knew how to have fun but took this job pretty seriously at times.

Another minute passed by and dispatch had an update for us. "Paramedic 2 and Fire, the RP is saying that she now has both hands trapped in the snake's mouth."

Holy shit, this sounds like it is getting interesting. Half a minute later: "Units responding to Pine Street, the snake is now wrapped up around the victim's arms."

I was starting to wonder how we were going to get this snake off. "Do we cut off its head, give it a shot of Versed, take it to the ER?" I asked Billy, but he didn't respond.

"Is there something wrong, Bill?" I asked.

"Nick, I don't like snakes — at all," he replied.

I told him not to worry, I could take this call.

I went into the house first and saw a woman with an albino python at least 12 feet long wrapped around both her arms. Fingers from both of her hands were trapped in the snake's mouth. Luckily, one of the firefighters had a degree in zoology and knew what to do. He grabbed the snake by its head and had a couple of us slowly unwind the body. I put my knife back in my pocket. Guess I didn't need to kill a perfectly good snake.

In my peripheral vision I saw Billy walk into the house and quickly out again. By the time we had only one coil left to unwrap, Billy had walked outside and then back into the house. Before we finished unwrapping, Billy had left the house again. Each time he did this he came in empty-handed. I didn't have a clue what he was doing. The firefighter was working on getting the patient's hands out of the snakes mouth when Billy came in for the last time.

"Fuck it, I'm out of here!" Billy swore, and with that he left the house and didn't come back in. He said it loud enough so everyone in the house could hear, including the patient. We put the huge snake back into the aquarium where it lived. We walked the patient to the ambulance when Billy apologized and said he could take care of the patient.

I jumped up front and listened to the woman tell her story. She had been feeding her son's snake a mouse when the snake struck her and caught two fingers on her right hand in its mouth. She called 911 and then tried to pry the snake's mouth open with the other hand, which ended up getting caught also. She was doing her best to yell to the 911 operator on the other end of the phone. The snake started to coil around her arms and then shortly after, we showed up.

Billy then told his story how he was terrified of snakes and confessed that it took every ounce of courage to go into the house the first time. He couldn't take it any longer and left. Twice more he came back in, only to freak out again and leave. Upon his final exit and comment, he didn't realize how loud he had spoken. The patient just laughed and said it was fine. She appreciated his attempt.

The woman ended up with three fractured fingers. She told her son she would not be taking care of the snake anymore. The snake was a little traumatized and did not eat for a while, but eventually went back to eating mice. Billy is still scared of snakes and I still laugh out loud when I remember the look on his face and hear the echo of "Fuck it, I'm out of here."

Chapter 13

Dead People Can Be Funny

By Nick Hoskin

While our job is often tense and serious, sometimes we laugh or joke to relieve tension. Sometimes a joke is just begging to be told. Other times things happen that are just too funny.

Imagine six guys (firefighters, police officers, my ambulance partner and me) standing around looking at a dead guy lying on his bed. He has been dead a good long while and there is nothing we can do — he's dead. For some reason, the lights won't work and trash and beer cans are littered everywhere. Just walking around the room, you can't help but kick a few beer cans. We are just looking at this guy on his bed that is by a window, making small talk and questioning why he died. We figured he drank himself to death.

All of a sudden the wind catches the curtains and billows them out. My partner, thinking the dead guy just moved, screams like a little schoolgirl. The rest of us start laughing so hard it hurts.

Chapter 14

Diabetic

By Nick Hoskin

It came down as just a routine diabetic call. You know—the patient is a little low on blood sugar, and the person who found him needs a little help. If the patient is still conscious enough, I will mix up a glass of juice with sugar to raise the blood sugar. I try to avoid IVs if I can because I feel it is better for the patient. This is just a personal preference.

On the day of this particular call, my partner, Jim, and I responded to a nice little house in a quiet bedroom community. A young woman in her early 20s met us at the door and said that her husband, Mike, who has diabetes, was in the bedroom and that she had been unable to get him to drink anything. She had checked his blood sugar less than five minutes before we had arrived, and it had been 31. Normal blood sugar is 80 to 120. A police officer had also shown up at about the time we did.

We went down the hall to a small bedroom. The wife sat on the bed at her husband's feet. The police officer was at the foot end of the bed, and my partner and I were at the side of the bed. The wife pointed to a glass of juice on the nightstand that her husband wouldn't drink. Jim gave it to the patient to try again. Our patient was just sitting there; he was awake and conscious but seemed out of it.

"Mike, my name is Jim," my partner said. "I'm a paramedic here to help you. Can you drink a little of this juice for me?"

"No," Mike responded, with a little more clarity than I was expecting.

"When was the last time your husband had an episode like this?" I asked Mike's wife.

"Probably about nine months ago," she told us. "He is usually good about managing his blood sugar."

"Nick, can you spike me a bag of saline," Jim said. "I'm going to start a IV and give him some D-50."

This seemed like a good idea to me. Sometimes it is just easier to start a line, give the patient a little sugar and wake him up that way. Even though Mike seemed coherent, his blood sugar was 31, which is low. From this point, it was only going to keep going down.

Jim pulled a tourniquet out of the kit and knelt on the bed to tie off Mike's arm so that he could start an IV. As soon as Jim leaned in, Mike took a huge round-house swing at Jim. Jim pulled back just enough so that Mike's fist only grazed his nose. Mike coiled up his legs and kicked his wife square in the chest;. That kick sent her flying into the arms of the cop, who was standing at the side of the bed. They went down to the floor. I dropped the IV bag I had just spiked and reached in to grab Mike's legs. Lucky for me, Jim was right on top of things and grabbed Mike's upper body. Together, we pulled our patient off the bed and onto the floor. Both Jim and I jumped on top of him and held him to the ground. For a little guy, Mike was putting up a good fight. I had got my knee buried in the side of Mike's leg — and that has to hurt — but he was still a handful.

"Hello, fire department, did someone call for an ambulance here?" came a voice from the front of the house.

"We're back in the back room," Jim yelled. "Get back here now. We need some help."

I was asking the officer for help, but he was still trying to untangle himself from the patient's wife. An EMT from the fire department walked in and held down the patient so Jim could start an IV.

I was still sitting on Mike's legs, and he was still trying to win this battle. Maybe somewhere in his mind he thought that this was a life-and-death struggle and that we were the bad guys. I asked the wife if she was OK. "Yeah, I'm fine," she said. "Just take care of my husband."

"I've got the IV," Jim said. "Pass me the D-50."

He pushed the dextrose through the IV line. Mike struggled less and less.

"Hey guys, how ya doing?" Mike said. "Oh shit, did my blood sugar drop again?" he asked.

"Yeah, we just did a glucose stick and got a reading and it was 22," Jim said.

"Oh man, I'm sorry. I hate it when this happens."

"The person you should apologize to is your wife," I told him. "You kicked her hard in the chest."

"No way. I'm so sorry, honey. Are you OK?" He spoke to his wife with real concern in his voice.

Mike seemed like he was back to his old self. His wife was doing fine, we'd checked his blood sugar, which was now 185, and his wife was going to get him something to eat. Mike didn't want to go the hospital. He has had this disease since he was a kid, and he knows how to take care of himself. He told us he forgot to eat because he became engrossed in a project for work. We pulled out the IV, filled out the appropriate paperwork, and headed out the door.

We walked back to the ambulance. "Jim," I said, "you are lucky that punch didn't connect. You'd have been the patient." We both laughed.

That was a fun call.

Chapter 15

Sights and Smells

By Nick Hoskin

Someday you will get one those calls that makes you want to puke, if you haven't already. I was reminded of my first "make-me-want-to-puke" calls yesterday when I transported a patient to the ER who thought she had an infection from an IV after a suicide attempt. We put her in a room right next to a guy whose lower leg was rotting from a true infection that had gone untreated. The smell was awful. I would think, given time and lack of care, our female patient may have ended up the same way as the guy in the next room. This made me glad I don't work in an ER.

Years ago, when I was a seasoned EMT with three years of experience under my belt, my partner and I went on a call for an elderly woman who fell from her bed and ended up just needing a lift assist. We arrived to find firefighters had already put the lady back into her bed. Walking into the house, I immediately noticed the heat. It must have been 90 degrees in there.

"Hello, paramedics," we called through the open front door. Fire said they were in the bedroom down the hall. As I walked into her bedroom, the smell of human feces assaulted my olfactory senses. I hate the smell of shit. I found the patient sitting in her bed, her underwear down around her ankles, and I noticed that one of her legs looked gimpy. She later said it was from a previous CVA (stroke). At the foot of the bed was one of the firefighters staring straight at her crotch. I don't know if this was intentional or not. He might have just been staring off into space not even paying attention to what he was looking at — after all, it was 3:00 in the morning.

It was my turn to attend, so I went up to the side of the bed and asked her if anything was wrong. She said "No, I just fell out of bed and couldn't get back by myself with my bum leg and all. I needed to go to the bathroom, and as you can see, I didn't quite make it."

I am doing everything in my power not to puke: breathing through my mouth, looking away, searching for a way to get out of here without being too unprofessional. The heat, the smell and the firefighter staring at her crotch was getting to be too much.

"Do you need help with anything else?" I asked.

"No, I have a friend coming over to help me clean up," she said. "You are so sweet to come and help, I hope I haven't been any trouble."

"Not at all ma'am, have a good rest of your night," I said as I pushed my way through the wall of stench and firefighters and sprinted to the door. She probably couldn't hear what I was saying because I said this as I was running out of the room. My partner was already waiting at the ambulance when I came out. I choked down the bile that was rising in my throat, a cold sweat covering my body, telling him, "That was fucking disgusting. I think I'm going to puke!" He just laughed; that smug laugh of a seasoned paramedic who knew enough to leave the room fast and let his EMT partner take care of this patient.

I started walking down the alley where we had parked to

get more fresh air. My partner followed in the ambulance making retching noises on the PA. I gagged a couple of more times as I heard this before I finally started to feel a little better. I was making $5.75 an hour and seriously questioning if it was worth it. I had been up and working for the past 20 hours, still feeling nauseous from smelling shit and seeing a dirty old fireman staring at an old lady's crotch. It wasn't the first time I questioned my choice of careers, and it wouldn't be my last.

Chapter 16

Oh, Gross!!!!!

By Lana Bond

One of the questions I get asked most often (particularly by new or aspiring EMTs) is, "What's the grossest call you've ever taken?"

Oh, the possibilities.

Generally, these glowing newbies are expecting a tale of blood-and-guts horror —"Entrails everywhere, I kid you not," and the like. Decapitations, hangings, decomposed bodies of the long-since deceased ...

Speaking of decomposed, the first DOA (dead on arrival) I ever encountered was during my field training. It was the first time I had ever smelled the odor of death. The call went out as "a possible code black (deceased) on a party not seen for about six days." The person in question had last spoken to his brother nearly a week before and reported that the man had been very depressed during the conversation. The brother became concerned when he couldn't reach the depressed party again. Eventually, the brother called 911.

We showed up on the lawn of a run-down apartment complex, where the police and fire and a small crowd of neighbors/onlookers (including the caller) had already gathered. The brother leaned against a tree looking nervous but at the same time as though he already knew the outcome of this venture.

The unseasonably hot evening of an unseasonably hot week shimmered against chipped paint of an uncertain color, and we sweated and waited for police and fire to find a way into the locked apartment. The man's body was visible from the windows by the door, but he was unresponsive and the fire department didn't want to break down the door. Eventually, a ladder was brought from the fire truck and propped against a west-facing window, and a stocky officer fumbled his way up. He forced out the window and then the screen.

The smell of the man's decomposing body crept out across the lawn and hit us like a physical slap in the face — bitter and dark and so very, very real. The smell of decaying human is unlike any other smell you will ever experience. It is unmistakable, even if you've never smelled it before. You'll never forget that smell, even if you never smell it again. Years later, you can draw it out of your memory like a bad dream. It is cold and greasy, sour but somehow raw and sweet, and disturbingly, distinctively human. It crawls into your hair and your skin and your nose and seeps into your clothes and your pores until it wafts out of your every movement. It clings to the back of your senses, and you'll smell it at odd times for days to come. It is the odor of raw meat and still blood and old bowels and dysfunction. It is distinctively different from the smell of dead animal. It leaves a residue on everything it blows past. The smell of a dead human is like a living thing in its tenacity.

I glanced at the brother whose still face had tightened into a mask of sickness and sadness and harsh reality, and I felt a wave of pity for him. It was the worst way for him to receive the news of his brother's death.

The paramedic on our ambulance took the monitor and left his partner and me standing in the yard.

"You don't need to see this," he told me. "You'll see plenty of this kind of thing."

When we asked him later how he thought the man had killed himself, he shook his head. "You couldn't tell," he said. "He might have shot himself in the head. He could have taken pills. There was enough black fluid coming out of his mouth and head that it could have been blood or vomit."

While that was one of the most disturbing experiences I have had, it really wasn't the grossest. That award would go to the time my partner and I were sent on a lift assist at a small, first-floor apartment in a middle-class suburban complex. We showed up with fire and found a mid-30s female who weighed in at well over 250 pounds. She was sitting on the floor, propped against a recliner. She was diabetic and had swollen legs with a chronic case of cellulitis. The cellulitis had progressed to a point where the skin was weeping a clear, meaty-smelling liquid, which had soaked into the carpet below her. On top of this, she had several cats, which were apparently throwing up cat food and hairballs on a fairly consistent basis and whose vomit the woman was unable to clean up due to her size.

As indicated by her call for help this night, once she got down she was unable to get herself back up. Puddles of cellulitis fluid and cat vomit spotted the floor and gave off a rank odor — not unlike vomit and litter box. We helped the woman back into her chair, avoiding the seeping skin of her legs as much as possible. We then offered politely to take her to the hospital to be checked (which she less than politely declined) and got the heck out of the apartment and into the fresh night air. Fire department and ambulance crews alike took a deep breath of air in an attempt to clean out the alveoli of our lungs. Cellulitis juice and cat puke. Words fail me …

While I was still in EMT school and did my very first ambulance ride, my crew was was sent to transfer a man from home to hospice. It was March, and the night was cool, but the house was stuffy and hot. The first thing to hit me was the smell. The smell of dogs, bile, and something akin to canned pea soup hit me upside the face with a wave of overheated air, and I immediately shut my mouth and began to draw short breaths in through my nose. I swallowed. The second thing to hit me was a noise that sounded like someone sucking the last few drops of a shake through a straw. It was rhythmic and repeated itself about every five seconds. Two large dogs trotted up and began industriously sniffing my boots as the ambulance crew and I made our way to a corner of the living room where a hospital bed was set up. In the bed, a skin-covered skeleton was lying on its side. A viscous fluid the color, consistency and odor of which was not all that dissimilar to the pea soup I thought I'd detected earlier was running out of his mouth and nose every time the man exhaled. Quietly and gently, the ambulance crew slid the man onto the stretcher and wheeled the man into the ambulance where I hopped into the back with the paramedic. He handed me a suction catheter and instructed me to suction out the man's airway. Because the man had a DNR (do not resuscitate), no further action could be taken to keep him from aspirating the fluid. As we got under way, the paramedic glanced at me over the top of his paperwork.

"Do you know what that stuff he's breathing is?"

I took a guess. "Bile?"

"Naw. That's diarrhea. Feces."

I blinked. The man was in the final stages of colon cancer. His digestive system had backed up to the point that everything in it — partially digested last meal and all — had come back up his throat and then been inhaled into his lungs. Every time he breathed in or out, more diarrhea ran into or out of him. Poo in the lungs. I swallowed hard. Incidentally, this particular call was the first turning point in this career for me. It was a moment where I could have backed away from the outstanding grossness of the situation or stepped up to really get my hands dirty (metaphorically speaking). I stepped up. And I hoped that I'd be able to keep stepping up.

Further on the weird end of the spectrum was a call I ran in a cheap trailer park. The call dropped for a mid-50s male who was "not feeling well."

Parties "not feeling well" can range anywhere from hypochondriacs who felt fine this morning and managed to talk themselves into the measles by the end of the day to healthy people who just want a check-up "just in case" to people about ready to drop over and go into cardiac arrest. We rolled up on a trailer with a small, tidy planting of flowers around the mailbox, and I hoped internally that this patient would actually need us, would have a real ailment. If the nicely maintained exterior of the trailer was any indication, this guy was pretty normal.

The moment we opened the door, any illusion of normality was shattered. Stacks of porn magazines as high as my waist were lying open everywhere. I lived a very sheltered life growing up, and the total extent of my exposure to porn until this point had been one episode of "Friends" where Joey and Chandler get free porn. Pretty tame. At first, I didn't quite realize what I was looking at. When I did, I tried to turn my eyes, away but it was everywhere! As we walked in, my partner nudged a magazine with the toe of his boot and discovered a very used looking dildo underneath. I found one section of carpet without a spread-eagled magazine on it. It was about 10 inches in diameter. Slightly off of center, a drying pile of porn reposed quietly beside a rock-climbing magazine left open to an ad with a scantily clad female climber. My heart sank. I'm a rock climber. I've even modeled for a climbing shoe manufacturer, and the idea of some weirdo jacking off to my photo in a sports magazine made me mildly nauseous. Across the room, a television show about ballroom dancing blared from the television set and three large jugs of Jack Daniels whiskey rested near a coffee table, also covered in pornography. And next to the coffee table, there was a vomit-colored sofa with a heavy-set, flushed-looking, middle-aged man upon it ... sans trousers. A damp-looking flannel shirt strained at the buttons over his belly and drooped down just far enough to cover everything I didn't want to see.

Regardless, I didn't know where to put my eyes. They darted from one item to the next as they sought a safe place, wanting not to see anything and yet somehow seeing everything. I sort of wanted to cry. But really I desperately wanted to laugh.

"I feel real sick," huffed the apparition before me, breathing heavily. There was a glistening coat of snot on his salt-and-pepper mustache. "I haven't been able to keep anything down but Jack and Coke for the last several days."

My partner rallied.

"Nothing at all? You haven't eaten anything?" he asked in a strangled voice.

"Well, I had a hot dog earlier today ..."

It was about 8:30 a.m.

"Let's ... let's go to the hospital," my partner said. The man stood in a heavy puff of odor. The smell of old sweat (very old sweat) mixed with the smells of old urine (*very* old urine), body grease, unwashed hair and the sour odor of old alcohol wafted into the air like oil from a deep-fat fryer and attached itself to the interior of my nostrils to haunt me for the remainder of my shift. I willed myself to smile at the man, and we loaded him up onto the pram. As we walked out to the ambulance, I shot my partner a pleading glance, and he very gallantly stepped up and offered to attend on this call. I crawled gratefully into the front of the ambulance and drove to the hospital, where we transferred our guy into the care of ED (emergency department) staff. He promptly vomited on the floor. Angry glances from nurses all around. Outside in the ambulance bay, my partner and I gasped with laughter as we decontaminated the ambulance and pram thoroughly with disinfectant wipes. We later discovered the man had an extensive psychiatric history. We weren't shocked.

EMS and grossness oftentimes go hand in hand. Contrary to common belief, though, the grossness doesn't often involve blood and guts and exposed bones or brain matter. More frequently, it's things like lifting a quadriplegic out of bed and finding her backside steeped in three days' worth of diarrhea or going to transfer a morbidly obese patient — obese to the point where the patient can't bathe or clean himself and, as a result, is full of the sweat, crumbs of food, and general filth of living that have gathered and rotted between the folds of fat. When the rolls of skin are disturbed, a very distinctive odor flows out and engulfs the room.

Gross is going to a fraternity and following a trail of poo logs down the stairs to the bathroom to find a teenage male, completely naked, passed out, face down in a pile of his own vomit — and he'd had a giant burrito for dinner. By the time you and the fire department get the inebriated youth to your ambulance, turds have been tracked all over the house. And the house isn't even his.

Gross is body fluids soaked into the carpet, animal by-products left unattended, genital infections, and that guy who walked himself into the ED with a gangrenous wound in his foot only to walk back out again after hearing that the foot would have to be removed, only to return a week later to agree to the amputation, only to return again three weeks after that with a recurrent infection. Gross is the fact that you can smell that foot from the hallway outside the ED, and when you walk into the ED, a nauseated-looking tech is spraying the air with wildflower air freshener and shaking his head. Gross is the photo shown you by the ED nurse of a foot so rotted away you can see the exposed muscle, tendons, and ligaments beneath. In EMS, gross is anything that can make your partner, who has 15 years of experience, who has seen it all, done it all, then seen and done it all again, grimace, gasp and say "That. Is. Gross!!"

Chapter 17

My Best Call Ever

By Nick Hoskin

It was mid-summer, a beautiful day to be working on the Front Range in Colorado. My partner and I had just run a double fatal motorcycle wreck up the canyon. A husband and wife had gone out for a ride on this beautiful day. They were wearing full leathers, helmets, the works. The canyon is a classic Colorado roadway that winds its way up the mountain on a curvy route that is surrounded by picturesque scenery. The creek spills its way down the mountainside. The couple was coming down and some other motorcyclist riding up the canyon crossed over the double yellow line. He hit them going around the corner.

This was the same corner we had been to a couple of weeks ago when another motorcyclist lost control of his crotch rocket. On that wreck the rider lost control of his bike and slid on the road and somehow his helmet got stuck under the metal railing. His momentum kept his body going; the helmet stayed where it was. X-rays showed about an inch gap between his first cervical vertebra and his skull. He survived a couple of hours till his heart realized it couldn't live with this kind of injury. Same corner as the wreck with the couple. Weird.

Fire was first on scene. Somebody had put a blanket over the husband. He was dead. His head was knocked off, held on by a piece of skin. My partner and myself were called with the fire department. When fire arrived on scene they called for a second ambulance for the guy who caused the accident by crossing the yellow line. He had a little knee pain, he might have had some drinks earlier. The paramedic with the fire department had intubated the wife and started a couple of IVs while his partners were doing CPR. I checked on the guy who hit these two, then on the wife who was being attended by firefighters and then finally on the guy under the blanket. As I was lifting up the blanket I questioned my own morbid curiosity. How was the coroner going to get this dude's head out of that helmet? To be honest, it kind of freaked me out.

The firefighters had done a good job, and the wife had a pulse and blood pressure. We loaded her into the back of our ambulance. Somehow we pulled out one of the IVs while doing this. Our patient had a heart rate in the 130s with weak radial pulses. The other ambulance had arrived by this time, and they were loading up the guy who caused this collision.

Going down the canyon, I started an EJ (external jugular IV) and continued to monitor her vitals. About five minutes before getting to the ER, she lost pulses. We started CPR again, dumped in more fluid to see if we could get anything back. Pulling into the bay at the hospital, we unloaded our patient. Somehow I pulled the EJ. This call sucked and it was just getting worse. Not that she had a real chance the minute her body hit the pavement. When you die from blunt trauma you have a 99 percent chance of staying dead. She was pronounced dead about 10 minutes later.

In my mind, I could still see her husband's dead eyes staring at nothing, his head sitting inside a helmet. The helmet did its job; his head was whole and safe.

I wasn't very hungry for lunch. My partner ordered a prime rib sandwich at a local sandwich shop. I ordered a smoothie and found even that hard to choke down. Right after lunch a tone dropped for a male party who had crashed while snowboarding up in the mountains. The area was up high, up near the Continental Divide. It is a beautiful area. If you go high enough there is snow year round. It took us about 35 minutes to drive there.

We parked our ambulance, took off our white shirts and grabbed our med kit and narcs (narcotics for pain) and headed in. We had about a six-mile hike ahead of us. It was glorious. Sunny, warm, the wildflowers were blooming, and nary a cloud in the sky. And to think we were getting paid for this. At some point, the fire department in this jurisdiction had called for a helicopter. It was on its way. We kept hiking. We must have been hiking for about two hours when we heard the sound of a chopper getting closer. It passed over our heads and rounded a bend. We kept on hiking. Twenty-five minutes later the helicopter passed over our head again heading east back to the flats.

We sat down and took a little rest. We had time to listen to the mountains. I had time to get some perspective. I could feel and smell the clean air. The trees were green and the sky a brilliant blue. Birds were flying around looking for things to eat. Life was good again.

The outdoors is my religion. That's part of the reason I moved to Colorado. I looked around, saw the beauty that is available in the mountains and felt renewed. I was still bummed about the motorcycle call, but somehow being out among the mountains and wildflowers and wilderness reminded me that life is good. It's death that sucks. Death sucks for the living. I don't think the dead care anymore. They're dead.

For me, one of the best things about working in Colorado is

going on calls where we have to hike in. This one was one of the best. I needed the physical exercise to work out some of the stress. I needed the beauty to remind me how great life can be and I needed to not work on any patients for a while.

Chapter 18

Pediatric Cardiac Arrest

By Nick Hoskin

"Stop CPR. Let me see the underlying rhythm," I say to the police officer who is doing compressions on the 6-month-old boy. This is not my first cardiac arrest. I have been on dozens before. However, it is my first pediatric cardiac arrest. And it sucks.

...

Dispatch airs: "Ambulance 41 and Fire, respond to 26 *Fencepost Way* for a baby not breathing." The tone dropped about 10 minutes ago.

"Paramedic 1 en route," my partner tells dispatch. My partner, John, and I head to the ambulance. I don't know how many times I've been called to "baby not breathing" only to have it be a kid who was choking on spit then coughed it out.

"Paramedic 1 and Fire, you're responding on 6-month-old male who is unconscious, CPR in progress," updated dispatch.

John drives like he is possessed. Three of the six wheels are off the ground going around the corners. My brain is going still faster than the ambulance. "Oh, shit, this is the real one," screams through my mind.

We can tell the house a couple of blocks away. There are at least four police cars with their doors open on either side of the street and in the lawn. We pull up. John slams the ambulance gearshift into park. We get our kit and heart monitor from the back of the ambulance.

One of the first things I notice is the mother outside near the front door wailing. "NOOOOOO … my baaaaaaby … NOOOOOO … AUGHHHHH!!!!" It is the kind of wail that goes right to your bones. It pierces your brain and your very soul. You don't have to have kids to hear and feel the pain of this mother.

When we walk in the house, we see a bedroom door open upstairs. Several cops are standing outside the door and in the bedroom. I don't know how many or whom, exactly. This thing happens to me on more serious calls — my line of vision narrows, it almost becomes tunnel vision. I pick up on a few things and focus.

In the room, one cop is performing CPR with the heel of his hand and the other cop is administering rescue breaths. As I kneel down, I tell John to get the kid on a heart monitor. I open the kit and pull out the pediatric ambu-bag. I start bagging the patient. His face is so small. It is easy to hold the face mask with one hand and ventilate with the other. I show the cop and tell him to continue doing it. In less than a minute, the fire department shows up. I see Stephanie walk into the room. She works for the fire department, and we are good friends. "Start bagging and hold onto this tube. Do not let it go," I tell her. I trust her work.

As I pull equipment out of the kit, I ask multiple questions: "When was he last seen?" "What's his medical history?" "How much does he weigh?" "Is he on any medications or allergic to any medications?" The dad is standing there, amazingly calm, and giving me the answers I need. It is interesting how people respond so differently in times of crisis. He seems opposite of his wife, who is hysterical.

I pull out a No. 3 endotracheal tube and the small laryngoscope. The only baby I had intubated is the practice one — the hard, little plastic head with its fat, plastic tongue. The blade from the laryngoscope slides easily into this real baby's small mouth, the vocal cords are right there. Using my right hand I slide the endotracheal tube between the vocal cords. "Where's the bag?" I ask as I look around. It was right beside me. It seems that everything is moving at a million miles an hour, yet barely moving at all.

Placing the bell of my stethoscope over the kid's belly, I squeeze the ambu-bag. Good, no bubbles. I listen over the lungs and hear good breath sounds in both lungs. John has the heart monitor on, which shows an asystolic rhythm. Flat line. The heart isn't doing anything.

John is trying to get an IV in the kid's arm. He is poking around without any luck. I grab the interosseous (IO) needle out of the kit and grab the kid's leg. One finger below the knee on the medial (inside) side of the leg, I swab it with an alcohol wipe. This is another thing I have never done on a child in real life. I've practiced on practice legs and chicken bones. The needle easily goes though the skin and baby fat. I keep pushing and turning the needle. It hits the bone. POP. It goes through the tibia, just like on the chicken bone. I hook up the bag of saline to the needle and open up the flow valve. Nothing happens. Shit.

I look quickly at his neck and arms. Then I grab another IO and do the same thing to the other leg. This time it works. "How much does he weigh?" I ask again.

His dad answers, "About eighteen pounds, last time we checked."

Quickly I do the math in my head: Eighteen divided by two, give or take. I convert pounds to kilograms and then multiply that by 0.1. This gives me the dosage of epinephrine I need to give him. It works out to 0.9 milligrams of epinephrine. I push this through the IV in the kid's leg. It goes in easily.

I look at the monitor. He is now in ventricular fibrillation. In my mind I am questioning what I should do now. I can hear multiple paramedic instructors at school say, "Don't worry about V-fib in kids, it never happens."

I need to defibrillate the kid — and quick! It is two to four joules per kilogram. Nine times two is 18. So I defibrillate at 20 joules. He goes into a sinus rhythm. He has a heartbeat. Momentarily I am at a loss.

"Now what?" I think. We give lidocaine for post V-fib, so I pull up the correct dosage of 1 milligram per kilogram, or 10 milligrams, and push this through the IV.

"Let's get going to the hospital," I tell everyone. *"Now."*

One good thing about the patient is that he is small. It is easy to carry him down the stairs to the back of the ambulance. I take two firefighters with me as we race off to the hospital. On the way there, I listen again to the breath sounds. I don't hear anything. I pull the tube and re-intubate him. Checking breath sounds again, they sound good.

I have time to readjust the first IO I tried. I find that it is working. This is good, because I like to have two IV lines for cardiac arrests.

The heart monitor tells me his heart rate is slowing down. It is 80 and getting slower. I gave him another 0.9 milligrams of epinephrine. His heart rate speeds up. I radio the hospital.

"This is Paramedic 1. We are coming in emergent with a 6-month-old repeat, 6-month-old male, who was in full cardiac arrest. He has a perfusion sinus rhythm above 100. There are pulses with this rhythm. He is intubated and has two IOs. We should be there in five minutes."

"Room 1," is the reply.

I go over the details again in my head to make sure I haven't forgotten anything. I am pretty sure I covered everything. We park under the hospital overhang and pull out the bed. The patient looks so small on such a big bed. He has tubes and lines sticking out of his body and patches all over him. We are met at the door by two nurses and the doc. I tell my story of what happened and what we have done. The patient is picked up and moved to the hospital bed. The hospital staff begins its work. The stress is high, the staff seems a little on edge. The stress level always seems to escalate when the sick patient is a kid. I know that is true for me, especially on this call.

My partner, the fire department, the police department and I have all done our jobs. We delivered this baby to the ER with a pulse and blood pressure. He is alive and holding his own. Now it is time to clean up. I have to write my report and head back to base, restock, regroup.

My partner and I discuss the call, making sure we didn't miss anything. We compare notes. I ask him who was there from the fire department and the police department because I want to write them a thank you letter. The truth is that the only people I remember being on this call were my partner, John, and Stephanie, from the fire department. Everyone else felt like fillers. On calls like that, I focus on the patient. I don't see the faces of the people I am working with, even when I try my best to widen my field of vision. My mind is too full, thinking too fast to process the stuff that I don't need to process. Who is there doesn't matter in times like that. What I do or don't do for the patient is what matters.

That night it is hard to get to sleep. I feel wired.

The baby was moved to Children's Hospital and died the next day. We did our best. We gave what we could. We gave him a chance.

Chapter 19

Epistaxis

"Paramedic 401, respond to an epistaxis," Kelly from our dispatch center told us.

Dave, the paramedic working with me, picked up the mic to respond and asked if there was any additional information.

"Paramedic 401, it's an epistaxis, a nosebleed," Kelly said with an exacerbated sigh full of knowledge and authority.

It must have taken 30 seconds for Dave to respond because he was laughing so hard.

"Dispatch, 401, do you have an address or something? We need to know where we are going."

"Oh yeah, it's 351 Main St.," she said sheepishly.

"401, we're en route," Dave responded.

Nothing else needs to be said.

Chapter 20

I See Dead People

By Nick Hoskin

I saw another one this morning. A dead person. She wasn't dead when we got there. She became dead after a few minutes of us being there. But like most dead people I see, it wasn't my fault. She would have died no matter what I did or didn't do. That's just the way it is.

This dead person was a woman who was driving a nifty little convertible down a double-lane highway. The truck she hit had moderate damage to the rear tires. Her car had major damage to the front end and driver's side door. The truck driver said this car started veering into his lane, and he moved over as far as he could. Not far enough. This lady wasn't wearing a seat belt. Don't know if that really mattered or not. She probably still would be dead. She might have been having a heart attack or something else that caused her to wreck in the first place.

I've been seeing dead people for a long time. Almost 20 years. The first few were a little creepy, but after a while I got used to them. In fact, it became sort of fun. Dead people were usually on the "good" calls. It becomes easy to distance myself, to dehumanize the person who just died. I would remember them for the day or maybe even a week and sometimes longer. I give them names so my partner knows who I am talking about. The *squished dude,* or the *headless motorcycle rider, burnt guy, frozen solid lady, stinky guy, the dude with bugs crawling in his eyes.* They all get names for the day, but most are soon forgotten. Some of them will stay with me for the rest of my life.

Whenever I drive or ride my bike up the canyon I think of the kid who fell 40-60 feet while he was rock climbing and hit a big rock. He was alive when we got there. The place he fell was close to town and close to the trail. It took us a few short minutes to get to him. He was lying face up, with his head down below his body on a steep hill. I made the short climb up the hill to find him this way. Some guy was standing on the rock above him with a climbing harness on. I told him to take it off. I took the harness from him, stepped through the place you put your legs, somehow managed to get my pants situated with all the crap I keep in my pockets and cinched it around my waist. Another climber was setting up an anchor rope so we could get to this guy safely. I had my partner double-check my knots before I rappelled off the side of the rock. My partner was a climber and I trusted him with my life. I clipped into a rope that *fallen guy* had been clipped into so he wouldn't fall any further. So there I am, hanging on this rope, working my way past him so I can start to assess what is going on with him. He was moaning and moving around. I had it in my head the minute I saw him that I was going to get a big line started and nasally intubate him.

It had been a really nice day. Our start time was 6 a.m. We ran a call in the morning that was nothing, then we did a stand-by for a fair in town. A nice sunny hot day, and people enjoying the late-summer weather. After the stand-by we were posted on The Hill. The Hill is where young people from the university hang out, shop and eat. It's a great place to watch people and look at the hotties that live in this town. I was finishing up a paper for a class I was taking that was due in a couple of days. I was four classes away from finishing a bachelor's degree that I started 20 years earlier. My partner was great. Dave and I had been partners almost a year and he had come a long way during the year. I could really trust him with the bigger calls. He had dreams of becoming a medic so he had been working hard. Not to mention he was younger and had a great eye for the hotties who were walking by. This allowed me to concentrate on my paper — he would inform me when to look up.

We received a call for a fallen climber up the canyon, and Dave knew right where it was because he loved to rock climb. We were there in less than five minutes, gathered our equipment and hit the trail. This sounded like a "good" call, meaning the climber fell quite a way and was still alive. We knew we would have to act fast to give him a chance. I called a "chopper go" because I wanted to get this guy to a trauma center fast. The local rescue group was on the way with a couple of members right on our heels. It seemed that this was a great day. A nice fair, some pretty women on the hill, and now this call. My partner was loving it. He had never been on a fallen climber.

My patient was moaning and somewhat combative. I lubed up the tube with lidocaine gel and slide it into his right nare (nostril). He sucked it down like a champ. I looked to my left and there was some mountain rescue guy saying he was IV certified and was putting a tourniquet on his arm. All I said was "go big or go home." He slid a 14-gauge IV into his AC like he does it all the time. I looked up at my partner, and he looked pretty pissed. Once back in the ambulance I learned the reason for that look — he felt useless standing eight feet above the patient not being able to do anything.

Things were going along pretty well, so I left my patient in charge of the mountain rescue EMT and they started to get him packaged up. They lifted him into the Stokes litter and pumped the air out of the bean bag that helps secure the patient and protect the cervical spine and back.

It seemed to be taking a long time to get this done, but I am sure in reality it only took a few minutes. It was probably like when someone passes out for 30 seconds but the family tells you he was out cold for two or three minutes. I heard the chopper coming in and felt good about what we had done up to this point. My concern was that as soon as we took the guy from the position he was in — head down and feet up — and flip him around to get him down the incline he would go into cardiac arrest. He was in an extreme Trendelenburg (legs raised above heart) and all the blood was in his head and core body, which was probably keeping him alive. He had stopped breathing on his own a while ago and we were now breathing for him with our ambu-bag. Just as the patient was being lowered down the hillside, the flight crew walked up to the scene. The rescue group flipped the guy around and laid him on the ground so we could reassess him. Sure as shit, he went into cardiac arrest. The flight crew hooked him up to their equipment and made sure everything was working. After listening to breath sounds and confirming the tube placement they pushed a couple rounds of drugs, but it was time to stop working him. He was dead. There was nothing else to be done. Put a sheet over him, call the coroner, walk back to the ambulance.

It was not a good walk. I was pissed. I hate it when people die on me. Especially when they are young. It's better when they are old, you have to die sometime. No one gets out of this game alive, as a good friend once told me. But this guy took all the right precautions. He wore a climbing helmet, I heard he took climbing lessons, and seemed to know what he was doing. He screwed up by falling and not setting his protection (climbing anchors that are suppose to hold you if you fall) well enough. Dave said he must not have secured that last piece of protection well and this started a chain reaction. That top piece pulls out and then the ones below pop out one by one, like a zipper. This allowed him to fall

all the way to the ground.

We head back to base. Both Dave and I are in pretty foul moods. Not as bad as the patient's family is going to be when they found out their son, brother, fiancé just died. After restocking our supplies and cleaning up we get a routine transfer from a nursing home to the ER. I call up Joe at dispatch and ask if he could assign another crew. He does. Joe is a good guy. Some of the other crews give us a hard time for not pulling our weight.

"It's just another dead dude," I hear someone say.

My only response is, "Fuck off."

I married later in life and now have two young kids, a boy and a girl. Having kids of my own has changed the game of paramedicine for me. Calls are now somebody's son or daughter, wife or husband, mother or father. Having this touch of reality has made being a paramedic a little harder. Some people outside the business may say this is good, that you need to know your patients are people. I haven't yet decided if this is good or not.

I know I love being a dad and a husband. I have developed a tendency to watch my kids playing and can almost see them get hit by a car or fall out of a tree and what they would look like mangled and broken. Or I see in my mind what they would look like if they had cancer and had to get chemo. It sucks. It sucks to even think these thoughts. It sucks sometimes to work on people whose bodies are broken into unnatural positions, legs and arms bent at impossible angles. It sucks to think that someone's mom just died or someone's kid just got killed by a drunk driver. It could be my kid, my wife. Sometimes it's all too fucking real.

I've seen too many dead people. Not nearly as many as

some people and way more than others. We all react a little differently when we see death. After a particularly hard day, I have a nice cold gin martini to celebrate my life and the lives of my family. Or I have a couple of beers, feel my emotions below the surface, feel like crying at the littlest thing and feel the anger as the kids don't listen to something I told them to do. Then I know the deaths and destruction do affect me. Then I know that I'm not immune to what I see and deal with. If it really bothers me, I talk with my wife about the call to get some of the hurt out. She used to be a paramedic so knows what I'm going through. She loves me even when I'm acting like a wuss and cry like a little schoolgirl.

Next morning I wake up, go to work, deal with it one call at a time. Seeing dead people can suck, but it also helps me appreciate the time I spend with my wife and kids a whole lot more. I often wonder who I would have become if I wasn't a paramedic. I can be jaded and cynical, controlling and moody. I know this comes from being a medic and seeing the stuff I've seen. I also know there are paramedics who may read this and think I'm a wuss for even feeling the way I do. We each deal with life a little differently. Overall, I enjoy my job and feel that I really do help people. Most of the time, calls are just calls and I am doing my job. Occasionally, the calls get to me and I have to deal with the emotions.

Chapter 21

Bad Dog!!

By Nick Hoskin

"I'm over here in the shed. I was bit on the leg. I'm not sure where the dog is," the delivery driver told my partner.

We were called to a dog bite and arrived first on scene. The police department was coming and we were supposed to wait for a "Code 4," which means everything is safe, but we decided to drive in and look around.

We were going to stay in the ambulance in case the dog was still around. The house was an older-style farmhouse sitting on the outskirts of town. I couldn't see another house from here. The delivery driver was in the shed, where she usually left packages. We drove past the shed and looked around for the dog. The gravel driveway ended, so we turned around and parked by the shed, which was 15-20 yards away from our parking spot. The owner showed up just before us and was looking for the dog.

PD showed up and parked closer to the house. The cop was a big dude, 6 feet, 2 inches tall. As he got out of his car, I saw him take his pepper spray out of its holster. He started walking toward us, looking around. As he got closer, he asked us if we had seen   the dog.

As the words were still leaving his mouth, I saw the dog for the first time. The dog was a German shepherd, and he was charging hard. Ears back, tail low, running fast, not making a sound — no barking, no growling, just a full-out sprint.

"There's the dog!" I yelled as I pointed.

The cop raised his left hand with the pepper spray. In the moment it took him to raise the can, the dog was about 20 feet away and closing fast. He pulled his .45 Glock from its holster and shot four times.

The cop had taken a step to his left, and the dog landed hard a couple of feet behind him right by the front wheel of our ambulance. My partner was on the radio to let dispatch know that shots had been fired.

The dog was seizing, his tongue hanging out, his left front leg bent awkwardly back. Twenty seconds later, he lay completely still. He won't be biting any more people now.

The owner who had just come around the corner was yelling. "You just killed my dog!" he screamed. "Why did you have to shoot him?"

"I didn't have a choice," the cop replied with some anger behind his words. "Why didn't you call him back?"

"He was such a good dog — he wouldn't have hurt you," cried the owner.

"He just bit the delivery driver in the leg," the cop retorted.

By this time, other police officers had shown up and taken control of the scene. They led the officer who had just shot the dog over to their cars. One of the other officers took the owner back by the shed to gather information. I checked out the delivery driver to see how she was doing. My partner was checking out the dog to make sure he was dead and see where he got shot.

The driver had puncture wounds to the back of her calf but didn't want to be taken to the ER by ambulance. She got a ride from her supervisor.

The cop who had shot the dog was visibly upset. His eyes were red, and I could tell that killing this dog had been hard on him.

I think the owner of the dog also could see that. He finally admitted that this was the third person the dog had bitten and he made a great watchdog for the place.

I was a little shaken up. It freaked me out a little to see this dog dying a couple of feet away from me. On the way back to base my partner told me the cop hit the dog with all four shots — one on the front leg, which broke the leg, and three body shots.

Damn good shooting.

Chapter 22

Step Back

By Nick Hoskin

One of the things I enjoy about being a paramedic is training, or being a field instructor. I especially enjoy training paramedic students. I credit this to all the great teachers and partners I had in the field as both an EMT and paramedic.

One of the most important things I teach these soon-to-be paramedics is getting along with the other EMS providers, especially the fire departments. I take pride in my ability to get along with firefighters, even when some calls get a little contentious. Over the years I have noticed how much ego and control comes into play in the field of emergency medicine.

I had been working with Shannon for a couple of weeks, and I was helping her focus on scene control. She was having a little trouble gaining control of scenes, finding that fine line between being in control and being overbearing. We discussed when to take control and when to let the scene run, while working with fire and sharing our knowledge. After all, we are there to treat the patients with the best possible care.

"Shannon," I explained. "The way I treat fire is that I will go into a scene and ask what is going on and let fire continue with what is going on, unless the patient is sick

107

and needs a more rapid intervention. It's being laid back, while still being in control. I will not yell unless something needs to get done right away, and it is not happening. My theory is that this way fire will know when you are serious and need to get things done."

"OK, Nick, I'll try to be more assertive, but not too much," Shannon replied with a smile.

Her opportunity came in a short time later. We were called to a 62-year-old female with chest pain. Fire beat us to scene by a good three or four minutes. We took our pram out of the back of the ambulance and wheeled it into a single-story house in a neighborhood that seemed full of elderly people. Outside the homes were nice-looking with manicured lawns, and the inside of this house was very tidy and neat. An elderly woman was sitting on the couch hooked up to the EKG monitor. The fire paramedic was kneeling on the floor talking with the patient and the fire EMT asked us, right when we walked in the room, if we had aspirin. The patient was close enough that I could see the monitor. From a distance, the rhythm looked fast and narrow, a SVT, or supra-ventricular rhythm. This is not a rhythm that requires aspirin.

Shannon walked up close to the patient and waited for the fire paramedic to fill her in. He ignored her and kept talking with the patient asking her if she was allergic to aspirin. Shannon looked at the patient and said, "Hi, my name is Shannon. What's yours?"

"STEP BACK, SHANNON," came out of the fire paramedic's mouth.

I was doing my best to give Shannon room to work and not feel crowded. I had to look over to be sure what I heard. Shannon was looking at the fire medic, awestruck. She wasn't sure she really heard what she heard.

"STEP BACK, SHANNON," he said again.

Shannon looked at me to see what to do. I waved her off as I folded my arms across my chest and leaned against the wall. Fire had just changed the rules. I have enough of my own pride that I wasn't going to play by their rules. The patient was now all theirs. The route they were taking wasn't the right one, but I was livid. I was hoping that this screwball of a medic would ask for help with the IV so I could tell Shannon to step back.

Despite being pissed off, I couldn't let the patient suffer because of some ignorant fire medic.

"That looks like an SVT to me, maybe a little Adenosine would be better than aspirin. If you slow the rate down, I'm sure she would feel better," I said to the fire medic.

He didn't even look up. He had his EMT partner start an IV and they pushed some Adenosine. Guess what? It worked. The patient's heart rate slowed down and she felt better.

The fire medic rode into the hospital with us. I was up front driving. After dropping off the patient, we went outside. I was ready to unload on this guy. That is when he apologized to Shannon. My angry, controlling side wanted to yell, to gain back the control that was lost. I still wanted to put that fire medic's ego in check, make sure this never happens again. Yet I decided to keep my mouth shut.

Whose ego was bigger?

Chapter 23

Reality Check

By Lana Bond

I can't sleep.

Sometimes the reality of what I do is more than I can bear.

I realized today that sometimes I am someone's last memory. I don't think I'm quite qualified for that responsibility. Today something in that realization made me set aside the report I was writing and ask the silent patient in front of me if there was anything I could do. All she wanted was to know "are we almost there yet?"

We were taking her to hospice to die.

There isn't much one can say to those who are dying and know it. They are no longer fighting. They know what is happening. And they've accepted it. Sometimes they joke about it. Sometimes they cry. Sometimes they are afraid. And sometimes they are silent. Their battle is over. There is nothing left to do but wait.

I realize that I am going to be one of their last memories. I want to be a good one, but what do I know?

Sometimes we are blindsided by our own mortality.

Sometimes a white night comes along in pitch black. When four o'clock in the morning rolls around and I am dog tired, but still can't sleep, all I can do is be grateful that I don't have to work tomorrow.

Chapter 24

We All Fall Down

By Lana Bond

An 82-year-old woman somewhere just cut her wrists.

Oh. It turns out she may not have cut her wrists. She has *potentially* cut her wrists. That's different. But still sad.

A call like this has the potential to be very intense or very mundane.

Perhaps the old woman is too weak to cut very deep and is bleeding very little.

Perhaps she is so desperate to finally end her life that she's found enough strength to cut her wrists to shreds.

Perhaps this is her only way out of life, out of the nursing home, out of never-ending cycles of illness, pain, boredom, and loneliness, each following one after another in an eternal pattern.

Perhaps she only wants attention, for someone to love her, to notice her, to see who she is — not just another elderly face or another common illness, but a woman who lived and felt and gave and accomplished.

Perhaps she wants someone to see her as Rosa (or Betsy or Maryanne or Florence), not as "the one with asthma" (or mrsa, Methicillin-resistant Staphylococcus aureus, or congestive heart failure or renal failure or cataracts), not as the one who needs a wheelchair (or hourly medication or soft foods only or dialysis appointments).

Maybe this woman wants somebody to get a sense of who she is.

Maybe this woman wants to get a sense of who she is.

I can't keep this up. This job will make me crazy. There are too many too much like me, too much like what I may become, too much like everything I want to avoid.

Death is rarely dignified. Growing old often less so.

People ask me about suicide calls: how do you decide who to treat? There is no question. We treat all of them. Even the ones who really tried. Even the ones who have succeeded but whose bodies don't know it yet. We have no choice.

Suicide is more complicated than you might think.

Suicide is easier than it should be.

This woman hasn't cut her wrists. At least not badly.

They are taking her to the hospital non-emergent, where staff members will seemingly treat her with care, then forget about her before the end of their shifts. For a few minutes, at least, she will *feel* as though someone still wants her to be alive, cares that she's not dead. This woman likely does not want to cause her own death. She just wants to not be invisible.

So much the better for her. Suicide is so much more difficult than it seems. So many people don't succeed.

It's a windy day. But at least the sun is shining.

Chapter 25

The Fat Medic

By Hunter Lewis

Developing as an EMT or a Paramedic is like learning motor skills as a child. Babe Ruth was a shitty hitter for some time as he developed his skill sets. People have differing natural abilities, and that is a factor with any skill. The Babe had more natural ability to hit a baseball hard than, say, someone with Down's Syndrome. He went on to hit 712 home runs while consuming nothing but hot dogs and alcohol.

This business is much the same. I sucked ass as an EMT when I started, because I had no clue what I was doing. The things you learn in a book are only about 5 percent of the job. The other 95 percent must be learned through experience. Perhaps I had a little bit more than an average level of intellect and natural ability, but when I started, I was a train wreck. I remember the first four or five months of my career, I kept thinking: "What if my partner doesn't know what to do, and I don't know what to do, either? It scared the shit out of me. I imagine that paramedics often have the same experience at some point or another, albeit to a lesser degree

Just like some kid with cerebral palsy probably sucks at baseball, some people just do not have the natural ability it takes to succeed as a good, or even a decent paramedic. It is sad, but the world is evolving into a place where people think they can be anything they want. That is bullshit. There needs to be less handholding and less pampering for inept idiots who have no business in certain professions. This brings me to one of the funniest, but sloppiest calls of my career.

In recent months, the organization I was working for had been having staffing problems, training problems, response time problems, basically all the problems you don't want an ambulance organization to have. Every time people would leave this glorious $9-an-hour job, they would hire another dozen idiots, and we were lucky if two out of 12 stayed more than a couple of months, and even luckier of one of the two was worth a shit. These people did not get the time in the field training program that they needed or deserved, and so we had crews getting lost, not knowing where the hell they were, taking forever to get places close by, not hearing the radios, all kinds of unacceptable problems. This was largely the fault of management, especially when field training officers would tell them that someone sucked or they were not ready to work alone. Management would then force the field training officers to send unqualified personnel out on their own because the company was so shorthanded. It was awful.

I had been working with a field instructor for some time, and we were getting frustrated with the lack of talent that the company had been hiring. I was appalled at the knowledge and skills of some of these paramedics, some of whom said they had worked as paramedics elsewhere for quite some time. Even worse, many of these new employees had been hired not by choice but due to a lack of options. Then they wanted us to make chardonnay out of shit, and it just wasn't happening.

We had a trainee, we will call her Kim. Kim was a beast of a girl, shaped like a tomato. She was about 5-foot-4 and weighed at least 200 pounds, probably closer to 250. Quick, nimble, efficient, and athletic are a few words that never collided in the same sentence with her name. She was put with us for a no-bull evaluation of her abilities. This was right up our alley. I am the first person happy to be brutally honest with my opinions about everything, even if it shatters someone's feelings, and my partner was right there with me.

Kim was with us for quite a few weeks. She repeatedly proved to us that she had no idea what she was doing. She could not run a scene, she could not triage, she could not handle multiple patients, she couldn't get anything done in the back of the ambulance, she didn't even know all of her drug dosages and their indications. I watched her almost make a patient's chest wall seize because she didn't know the proper procedure for administering pain medication. If I hadn't questioned what she was doing, she probably would have killed this poor guy. Don't you want this idiot taking care of you when you are really sick?

Although Kim showed us that she couldn't really even run a basic call with any proficiency, she got her share of acute calls, which she consistently screwed up. One afternoon we got a call for an unconscious man sitting in a car. It was early fall, so it was still plenty warm out. We pull up to find a man roughly 6-foot-3, and he is fat. I would estimate that he weighed about 275 pounds. He was so sweaty that he was slippery, and he was snoring like a bear. We suggested that Kim start an assessment. She asked the fire department to help her get the man out of the car onto the bed. Other firefighters looked through the car for indications of what might be going on. After running lots and lots of calls like this, you can usually examine the situation quickly, and narrow your diagnosis to about three or four things. Not Kim. We had to tell her to do every damned thing. She was freaking out that this guy was breathing slowly with snoring respirations, and before she had done any evaluation at all, she was asking me to prepare for her to intubate him. It was the first quarter and she wanted to throw the Hail Mary. We fought off laughter. I calmly suggested that we check a couple of quick things that were far less intrusive first.

With a large, sweaty unconscious patient that is having a hard time controlling his airway, it is not a bad idea to check a few very basic things. For example, pinpoint pupils might be indicative of a narcotics overdose. We carry a medication that is used specifically to reverse a narcotics overdose, and we don't have to stick a tube in someone's throat to correct the problem. Likewise with checking a blood sugar. Diabetics have a difficult time controlling their sugar levels sometimes, but even if someone's sugar goes so low that they become unconscious, it is a pretty simple problem to correct with just some sugar through an IV. Besides, if you bring an unconscious person into the ER without a blood glucose check, and that turns out to be the problem, you are going to catch hell from all different directions. Everyone will make fun of you, and the attending physician might even punch you in the side of the head. I wish he had punched Kim, even though I had her check this guy's sugar.

Anyhoo, since it never occurred in Kim's genius mind to do some of these very basic procedures, I prompted her. The entire time, Kim was sweating like a whore in church, and my partner was just laughing. Blood sugar? Normal. Pupils? Pinpoint. Okey dokey. We have a winner. I next asked Kim what she would like to do. (I assumed she knew what pinpoint pupils likely indicated, but hey, I had to give her the benefit of the doubt sometime.) I asked her how much Narcan (the medication that reverses a narcotic overdose) she wanted to give. The idea with Narcan is to give the patient enough so that they begin to breathe more normally and regain SOME consciousness. You want to inhibit the overdose, but you want to keep them really lethargic. If you pull them all the way out of it, you have a junkie that is pissed at you for ruining their high. Recall that this guy was at least 250 pounds. If I hadn't told Kim to give this guy one-fourth of the dose she wanted to give him, we may have hosted a battle royale in the back of the ambulance. It is also worth mentioning that it is a good idea to tie this type of patient down before you give the Narcan. Usually, the seatbelts on the bed and a couple of wrist wraps suffice. Errant fists from a man 100 pounds larger than I am do not sound like fun, especially if they collide with my head. Do you think it occurred to Kim to tie the patient's hands and body down? If you said yes, you need to put this book down and go seek another profession. Once again, I prompted her that this needed to be done before anything else, and all my partner could do was stand at the back of the ambulance laughing. With the fire brigade. As a paramedic, if you are being laughed at by your field instructor and a bunch of damned firefighters, you have made at least one very large, obvious fuck-up in the very recent past. In this case, Kim had made about half a dozen, so my partner and the peanut gallery had their pick on which mistake to ridicule. Fortunately, yours truly was there to point it out on every single occasion. Nobody told me that it was "come feel better about yourself" day, but for my partner and me … it was.

So after holding her hand held through extrication, initial impression, size-up, assessment, plan of action, and part of treatment, our little beer keg-shaped protégé had done absolutely nothing on her own, and had almost made a number of mistakes that could have been called catastrophic. Fortunately, since we walked her through this very basic narcotic overdose call, all she really had to do was give a little bit of Narcan (because I started the IV for her) and take some vitals on the way to the hospital. I don't really remember, but she probably fucked up her radio report on the way to the hospital, too. If she did, it definitely wasn't the first time. I think it was after this call that my partner informed her she was "a shitty paramedic."

She cried for a little while, but who cares. It was true.

When I started this job years ago, I remember a couple of senior medics told me to pay attention and work hard because one day I would be "paramedic sitting." I chuckled at the time, thinking they were kidding since paramedics know way more than me. Years later, this call happened. They were right, and all I could think about was what a jackass I must have looked like, laughing when they told me that.

Editor's note:

When asking people to write stories, I asked them not to be politically correct, but to tell it like they saw it. The reason for this is a story just like this. This is a small look at what life can be like in the field. This is not to say all field instruction will be like this, but occasionally it does happen. There can be very little room for mistakes, and some field instructors are much less forgiving than others. I want to remind you that this is just one person's story, one person's opinion of one paramedic's experience while going through a training process.

Chapter 26

The Puke Story

By Hunter Lewis

The ambulance business is funny sometimes. Some people call it luck. Some people call it karma. Others think it is the will of God or some other religious justification they use for what went wrong. There are times when you as the paramedic can do no wrong — even when you don't perform perfectly, the call ends well and you hit home runs. There are times when you do everything absolutely perfectly, yet the call still ends poorly. There are calls that are neither serious nor easy, but for some reason just seem to go smoothly. Then there are calls that from start to finish are a complete shit storm.

Regardless of the outcome, it boils down to your ability to learn from the call, improve your skills, and ultimately look back and laugh. This is one of the characteristics that differentiates a good medic from a great one.

The following is one of those calls that was a cluster from start to finish:

It was the dead of summer, and it was very hot. We had been running lots of heat exhaustion and dehydration calls for several weeks. Wearing navy duty pants and a woven polyester uniform shirt with a navy blue undershirt didn't help. We could have just as easily worn form-fitting ponchos that didn't breathe at all. It was early afternoon,

119

the sun was beating down on the ambulance, and it was all the air conditioning could do to keep us cool. There was no breeze at all, and it was flat miserable outside.

We got toned to an unconscious party. My partner Hank grumbled at the radio because even an 80-degree ambulance is better than 97-degree outdoor heat. We arrived at a run-down apartment building, got the cot out, and put our jump kit and heart monitor on top. I was sweating profusely walking downhill on a concrete sidewalk. The police showed us into the patient's apartment. It was hotter in the damned apartment than it was outside, and it was stuffy. The apartment was a dirty wreck and smelled like cigarettes and filth. I was pissed. This is the kind of environment that I despise working in more than any other. People who don't take care of themselves and then expect us to come in and rescue them — it just doesn't make sense. On top of that, the patient was a fat woman, and because of the hot conditions, she was sweating like you wouldn't believe. This woman was the kind of big person who sweats when she peels an orange or brushes her teeth, but in this case it looked like she had been jumping rope in a sauna. Working on people who are really sweaty is gross, especially when they are completely dead weight. Anytime you're doing this kind of work, you're wearing rubber gloves and the patient ends up sliding around in your hands like a damned baby seal.

The patient was in her 40s. I could tell by looking both at her and around her living space that she had not taken very good care of herself over the years. She was completely unresponsive. I could have cut her enormous fat leg off with a dull, rusty butter knife, and she wouldn't have even flinched. She was having a difficult time maintaining her own airway, snoring loudly with erratic breathing patterns. Her blood pressure was low, and her pulse was fast and weak.

We decided that we would be able to care for her much more effectively in the back of the ambulance, plus her heat exhaustion would likely not improve in a 100-degree apartment. At this point, it looked like this call was going to suck no matter what. Perhaps it would suck slightly less, I thought, if we were working in the comfort of an air-conditioned vehicle.

With the help of the fire brigade, we got the patient into the back of the ambulance. While I worked at getting an IV into the patient, Hank noticed that the patient's snoring respirations were getting worse and that she was not maintaining her airway adequately. We decided that it was appropriate to nasally intubate her and assist her in breathing. I prepped the tube for Hank and put the patient into an upright sitting position. In case you have never seen someone get a giant tube shoved down her nose into her trachea, let me tell you, it is a sight to see. Some finesse is required to make the tube go down, yet somehow it still seems like a brutal process. Noses bleed, and because of a delightful phenomenon called the gag reflex, vomiting is not uncommon either. So here we were, huddled over a giant fat woman who was snoring so hard it sounded like a damned chainsaw, in the back of a tiny van, and it was heating up like an oven. I positioned her head while Hank started to insert the tube. As my luck would have it, she didn't like having a tube in her nose.

As I mentioned earlier, the patient had been completely unresponsive. Unfortunately for Hank and me, her gag reflex was not. She began vomiting. *A lot.* There was no dry heaving involved in this incident. It was like someone had turned on a hose. Not only was puke spewing out of her mouth, it was also filling her breathing tube. Since this indicated that the tube was not placed correctly, we withdrew the tube and tried again. Karma reared its ugly head at this moment, and although this giant woman no longer had a tube in her throat, she felt she had not yet puked enough. Copious amounts of vomit oozed and sprayed out of her mouth, puddling on her chest and stomach, splashing all over the Plexiglas cabinets, and splattering on the floor of the ambulance and my boots. I can't give a specific amount of vomit that emerged from the woman's stomach, but it was like she had just finished Thanksgiving Dinner.

All of this happened so fast that I don't recall our exact dialogue, but it probably sounded something like this:

Me: Oh, shit, she's puking.

Hank: Damn it. Oh … oohhhh, shit.

Me: The tube is in her belly. It's no good. Pull it.

Hank: Shit. She's still puking.

Me: Yep, she is sharing with the cabinets and the floor. How thoughtful.

Hank: What a mess!

Me: This could take a while…..

Finally, she stopped puking. She either got tired from retching or the tank ran empty. Either way, both Hank and I breathed a sigh of relief and prepared to intubate her again. This time, we were able to place the tube correctly without the woman hurling again. Thank God for small favors.

While Hank secured his handiwork, I looked around at the wake of destruction that this woman had created. It was everywhere. Every surface within a few feet of this woman's head had vomit on it. Cabinets, the cot, the floor, my pants and boots, my stethoscope — everything. We asked a firefighter to ventilate the patient so that Hank could clean up and complete some treatments on the way to the hospital.

When we got to the hospital, we took the woman into one of the rooms where the sickest ambulance patients start. Her body temperature was 104.3, which is very, very high, especially for an adult. Curious as I was about what was going to happen to her, I had other rats to kill. The ambulances don't clean themselves, so we get to enjoy doing it.

Cleaning the back of an ambulance is a real adventure. Your mind wanders about all the fucked-up stuff that has happened back there, and no matter what anyone tells you, it is impossible to have a perfectly clean ambulance unless it has never been used before. This woman had made such a horrific mess that I wasn't even about to bother with the little baby wipes we usually use to clean up piss and the stench of homeless people. This scouring required more drastic measures.

I have cleaned some filthy things. A mechanic's shop, dog pens — hell, I've even cleaned a god-damned fraternity house bathroom. That experience can change the way a person looks at the world. However, none of these things rivaled the task of cleaning this ambulance. I have scrubbed blood, brain matter, just about everything you can imagine finding in the back of a seasoned ambulance. Even the worst messes I have dealt with were nothing a mop and bucket and a bottle of 409 couldn't handle. Not this one. Not this mess. This was far beyond that. Fortunately, I was able to recruit a couple of newbies to help me with the mess.

As I was tackling the cleanup, the fire brigade had arrived to pick up the firefighter who had ridden with us. What ensued was at least a first for me, and none of the firefighters had ever seen it either. I asked if I could run a section of fire hose from the tank on the fire truck to the back of the ambulance to spray all the mess out. They all looked at me like I was joking. They started to laugh, until they realized I was completely serious. While some might think this technique was a bit of overkill, like killing a mosquito with a bazooka, I found that it worked beautifully. It pushed all that terrible, lumpy vomit out the back of the car. It cleaned the Plexiglas like a car wash. Sure a little water got in the cabinets, but I wasn't about to mop that shit up with Q-tips. After I had sprayed the majority of the mess out, all it took to make the ambulance at least usable were a mop, a towel, and some baby wipes. It didn't smell like potpourri in the back, but then again, it hadn't smelled that sweet when we'd gotten in it that morning either.

Exhausted from the heat and frustrated with the events of the day, the end of our shift could not come soon enough. I didn't bother to follow up on what happened to this woman, frankly because I was so pissed about the mess she made that I really didn't give a shit. When we got back to headquarters and got our belongings out of the ambulance, I found something to change into in the car and took off my disgusting clothes. It was so bad that I even wore rubber gloves to take my boots off. I put my clothes in a trash bag and made sure they didn't touch my skin until they had been through the wash. As I headed for home, I remember thinking to myself, "If that kind of thing never, ever happened to me again, I would be just fine with it. That sucked." Did I forget to mention that we do all this shit for about nine bucks an hour? Well, we do.

I went home and took a long shower. I remember scrubbing myself like a rape victim to make sure I didn't miss any trace of the wretched substance that had blessed us earlier in the day.

I thought to myself: When I wake up in the morning, I'll get to do it again.

Chapter 27

Shannon's Story

By Shannon Pringle

I once read that "storytellers are themselves a part of the story and not mere relayers of reality."

I want to tell you of a journey that began almost a decade ago. My story begins when I was 18 years old, when a friend and I were headed home from a show. We had made plans to meet up with some other friends who were home from college for the holidays. As we drove west on a two-lane highway, I couldn't help but admire and enjoy the beautiful sun setting behind the mountains. I remember vaguely that it was one of the most beautiful sunsets I had ever seen, with the colors of yellow and burnt orange so vibrant.

The next thing I knew I saw an angel at my car door. Two days later, I woke up in ICU at Denver General. I wasn't clear on exactly how I got there, but I was lying in a hospital bed, unable to move the right side of my body. As I lay there, I tried to forget about the pain but couldn't. All I could remember was the angel who had been at my side.

I asked what had happened, and my mother explained to me that I had been in a bad car accident. She told me that I was going to be OK but that I would need to have surgery on my right arm and leg. I ended up staying in the hospital for a month and having six surgeries.

As I look back on that hospital day, it seems to me like a weird dream. I have only vague memories of the events that took place during my stay. The doctors and nurses kept me reasonably comfortable with morphine pumps and oral meds, so I didn't really care what was happening. It seemed that I had reverted back to infancy. All I could do was lie there, slipping in and out of drug-induced sedations while others would come in and out of the room to take care of me, feed me, reposition me, bathe me, medicate me, help me use the bathroom, keep me company.

I would try to entertain my guests, but what I had to offer was a whole new kind of entertainment. I would push the morphine pump, and as the button pushed in, it would sound like I had pushed the button on *Jeopardy!* My sister would respond with, "Pharmaceuticals for $500, please." There always seemed to be constant chuckles mixed with tears. Yet the overall environment at Denver Health was one that was filled with love and admiration for the ones who put me back together. The statement that laughter is therapy couldn't have proved to be any truer. My family always knew how to make me laugh even when it hurt and at times when I didn't want to laugh.

The entire experience was quite humbling, and I am so appreciative of everyone who attended to my needs. When I was released from Denver General, I left with a completely new perspective and respect for life, as well as deep admiration for those who serve in the medical field.

It has almost been about nine years since the day of my car accident. I must say that I am thankful that it happened. I greatly appreciate all that I have gained and lost through the experience. It has allowed me to see life and the love for family and friends in a whole new light. It has also given me a new direction and determination to succeed in all I do, even though the thumb on my right hand is no longer functioning, it was somehow worth it.

The direction and determination that I speak of is pursuing and finding a new love for medicine. I wasn't sure after getting out of the hospital what direction within the field of medicine I was going to take, but I knew that I was intrigued and inspired by it. Since the accident, I've had 23 surgeries and have seen the doctors frequently. After I got out of the hospital, I saw the docs at least once a week and eventually was able to slow down to seeing them just once a month. Having spent so much time with doctors and others in the medical profession, my interests were piqued by all that they could do.

What caught my mind was how amazing the human body is. For example, did you know that doctors can sew your hand to your groin for two weeks just so they can replace the webbed space between the thumb and index finger? This procedure is called a groin flap. And did you know that they use breast implants (tissue expanders) to create ports? These are used to expand or stretch the surrounding tissue. Doctors used this method on me for cosmetic reasons as I had a chicken mesh skin graft just below my elbow that they wanted to replace. People always asked what happened to my arm and instead of going in to a long drawn-out conversation, I would respond, "I was bitten by a shark." By the looks of the graft, it must have been pretty convincing. The "breast implants" were placed in my arm, and I would go in two times a month to have saline injected into them via the ports until the skin was not able to stretch anymore. The other miraculous procedures included bone graft, skin grafts, and odd metal contraptions. These are only a few examples of what doctors can do and the contributing reasons behind my interest in the field of medicine.

But though I knew I wanted to pursue a career in medicine, I constantly asked myself three questions: "Where do I begin? Am I cut out for the medical field? *Why* do I want to do this?" After all, I had been the type of high school students who cared mostly about sports and did just what was required to get by in her classes. Plus, I wasn't sure how I was going to handle the blood and guts of it all. As I wondered why I wanted to do this so badly, the only answer I could find was that I wanted to give back what I had been given.

I decided to start small. I began with baby steps, and like a child, I grew stronger legs and was able to run with it in the end. My introduction to medicine was via the Radiology Department where I worked in the clerical area for a few years. My heart was inspired but still felt unfed. I found myself looking in other areas so I could learn more about medicine. I took a job working as an assistant tech in ultrasound for two years. Although I learned a great deal from this wonderful experience, I still felt this hunger and cry to do something more.

A good friend of mine shared this desire and hunger to do something more. Together, we found a summer EMT program at Front Range Community College. We enrolled and had one of the greatest summers of our lives. My friend went on to work in a cardiac cath lab, and I went on to work on an ambulance and in an ER. Looking back at how far we have both come, we chuckle and wonder how we ever got here. Together, we have found the one thing that continues to feed our hearts and that is helping those who are in need of medical attention.

My past experiences have definitely made me a better person and have allowed me to learn more about myself than I may have wanted to learn. These experiences have also made me realize that we all go through certain things in life, good or bad, for a reason. The hardest part about this whole thing is that we may never know the why behind the reasoning.

Chapter 28

Buzz Kill

By Nick Hoskin

It was Christmas Eve. I had Christmas Eve and Christmas Day off. This holiday has gained a little more importance for me since having kids, so I was really looking forward to a fun, annual Christmas Eve celebration with my sister's family and my own. Plus, a huge snowstorm had hit Colorado a few days earlier, so we were having a white Christmas for the first time in several years.

So, not only were there 20 inches of snow on the ground, but my mother, who usually spends Christmas with my younger sister on the East Coast, ended up being in town with us this year. All of the airline flights had been canceled in and out of Denver indefinitely. And to top it off, the Denver Broncos were playing the Cincinnati Bengals in a game to get into the playoffs. Since I grew up in Cincinnati and was now living close to Denver, I couldn't lose. I could only have fun!

It was a good first half, and the margaritas and beers were tasting good. At halftime we went outside to play a quick game of football. It was one of those crazy games in which you have a little buzz going from the drinks, it's cold and snowy, and we had to play in the street because the yard had two feet of snow covering it. The streets weren't much better. Big ruts of ice not only hindered the cars but made it a little difficult to run. Alcohol seemed to level the playing field out. We all sucked except for my nephew, who was 17 and hadn't been drinking. He made a beautiful catch by muscling me out of the way and diving into a snow drift. It was beautiful. The game was a blast and no one got hurt. There was still another half of football and a night of Christmas Eve celebrations to look forward to.

The game on TV was a lot of fun. I ended up rooting for the Broncos since they won. Two of the people who had come to watch the game headed for home. A little later my wife and kids showed up, and then my Mom showed up. Water was heating up on the stove for the shrimp we have each Christmas Eve. Dinner preparations were just getting under way. I was sipping a margarita in the TV room when my older sister yelled for me. "Nick, Mom needs you — now."

My first reaction was wondering what Sarah was overreacting to this time. She has a habit of getting a little excited at some things. That thought quickly passed as I heard the seriousness in her voice. Being a paramedic, I am often called when family members are hurt; usually it is one of the kids needs a splinter removed or advice on some kind of "owey." This time I could tell it was a little more serious than a splinter.

As I entered the room I saw my 72-year-old mother lying on the floor unconscious.

"Call 911 and get an ambulance for her now," I yelled. Within the short walk across the living room, I transformed from a slightly inebriated football fan into a paramedic. I was now in charge, I was in control of the scene.

"What happened?"

One of our friends, George, said she was starting to sit on the ottoman and it slipped out from under her and she fell and hit her head. I grabbed my Mom's head and held C-spine. Her eyes were open and I saw the look of someone who is dead. She had the *dead fish eye look.*

"Mom, wake up, can you hear me?"

No response.

"Does she have a pulse?" I asked.

Another friend, Charlie said, "Yeah, it's in the 80s."

Charlie had some medical training in the army a long time ago, so I trusted he knew what to do. At work, I trust my partner to give me the correct information.

I put my cheek down by her mouth.

Oh god, she's not breathing.

Two quick breaths.

Feel for a pulse, not sure if I feel one. She coughs and starts to move. My wife is off to my right, my 2–year-old daughter is sitting by her grandmother's head looking like she knows what is going on and is perfectly content to sit there while her Nana is unconscious on the floor.

"Is the ambulance coming?" I ask.

My nephew, who had an hour or two earlier schooled me in football, said the ambulance should be there soon.

My mom was doing better.

"What happened?" my mom asked.

"You slipped and fell, hit your head, and you were knocked out," I replied. "I'm holding your head in case you have a neck injury, does your neck hurt?"

"No, it feels fine," she replied.

I noticed that she had been incontinent of urine. Her pants were wet. She knew where she was and what day it was. My wife had gone off to take care of some of the kids who seemed a little shaken up. It seemed like it had been a long time since we called 911, and I was wondering where the fire department was and where the ambulance was. I also knew the roads were bad — I had been driving with chains on my ambulance for the past week.

After more time elapsed and I had time to check her out more thoroughly, I cleared my mom's C-spine (meaning I wasn't worried that she had a cervical spine injury). I had her sit up and at that time the fire department showed up. I saw Sara, an EMT and fire lieutenant whom I have known for years. I focused in on her, told her what was going on. I asked them to get me a blood pressure and gave them a synopsis of what had happened. I was clearly in charge, playing the paramedic I had been for years. I continued making decisions and getting things done.

I called up dispatch to slow the ambulance down to non-emergent because my mom didn't seem hurt. Then I went outside looking for the ambulance, wondering why they were taking so long. I went back inside to find out if anything had changed. Nothing had, except she was feeling a little better and that her left knee hurt. Finally the ambulance showed up, and the paramedic asked me what was going on. I told him the story I knew up to this point and that I had made the decision that my Mom was doing better and didn't need an ambulance and we would take her to the hospital by private vehicle. The paramedic was fine with that and ended up leaving. They parked the ambulance at the end of the road because they had gotten stuck so they needed to go get unstuck.

My sister and I walked my Mom to the car and started driving to the hospital. The hospital was about two miles away and didn't take long to get there. On the way out of the driveway we saw the firefighters pushing the ambulance out of the ruts so they could leave. I was still in paramedic mode, still in charge.

Arriving at the ER, I went in, grabbed a wheelchair and helped my Mom get into it so I could wheel her inside. I told the triage nurse what had happened. She took vitals and she got a pressure of 178/94 and a pulse of 46.

"Hmm, that's weird," I thought.

They took her back into Room 4 and hooked her up to a monitor and ordered a 12-lead EKG. I heard Michelle, a part-time EMT and paramedic student, talking to my mom's nurse about a syncopal. Clunk. Another piece of reality fell into place.

My mom had a syncopal episode, most likely due to having a bradycardic rhythm (slow heart rate). All this time I thought she had slipped for some reason and hit her head. I had not screwed up a call this bad in a long, long time. Of course I don't show up to calls all liquored up after drinking for the last few hours, and I usually don't have to run on calls that involve my loved ones. Luckily, I liked and trusted the doc who was working. He did all the right stuff.

Me, I was feeling like a complete dumb shit. We had been in the ER for 20 minutes or so and I was ready to leave. My sister couldn't believe that I wanted to leave. I couldn't see why I should stay. My work was done, done poorly, but it was done. I had delivered the patient to the hospital and it was time to depart, get ready for the next call or, in this case, go eat shrimp and drink margaritas. I knew this was wrong of me, I knew I had to stay, but I didn't want to. I went from having a great time, looking forward to a fantastic evening to having to be a paramedic and giving my mom two rescue breaths. I could still picture her dead fish eyes staring at me. The last hour had been a buzz kill, a big one. It sucked.

I never stay at the hospital very long. Drop off the patient, give the report, chat with some of the nurses and doctors and then leave, get ready for the next call. And here I am stuck, not really in a position to leave. My mom is still here, and I would get a DUI for driving. What a crappy Christmas Eve.

What I learned from this is to let the people working do the job they know how to do. I should have done what needed to be done in the moment but then let go of that control, let the fire department and my friends on the ambulance do their job. What I learned is that as a paramedic I will at times make a lot of decisions very fast. Most of the time they are good or if they aren't, I can correct them after I have more data. When this happened to my mom, I went from being at a family holiday party to becoming a paramedic in the short walk across the room — my buzz was gone, and my mom looked like she was dead. I made decisions that turned out not to be life threatening, but they were still not good choices. This haunted me for weeks after. I repeatedly asked my wife if I needed to give rescue breaths. Was she really that sick?

The next week was challenging also. Even without having alcohol on board I found it hard to make good decisions to help my mom. My wife, who used to be a paramedic, seemed to be able to make much better decisions when it came to my mom.

If the situation arises where I have to give medical aid to a family member, hopefully I will have the awareness to let the medical professionals do their jobs. That's what I do for people when I am working — help them make good decisions. But who am I kidding? I am a paramedic who is like most paramedics — controlling — and think that I know what is best, even when I really don't. Will I be able to let go of that control if this or something similar were to happen? Would I be able to trust the paramedic who steps out of the ambulance? I am going to guess it depends on who steps out of the ambulance and what is going on. If this happens again, I hope I will make better choices.

Chapter 29

15

By Lana Bond

The girl wore a denim, peasant-style skirt with a white tank top and sandals the day she died. She had a tattoo just above her pubis that stated "exit only" and one on the small of her back that said "entrance only," each with an arrow pointing down. Her mother called the police that day, saying, "My daughter is suicidal. Please help."

As the police stood in the living room and spoke with her mother, the girl took a pistol, placed it to her temple and fired. Police heard a pop in the next room. They found her with a hole in her head and the gun between her knees. She was still breathing.

As we pulled up to the house, fire was already carrying the girl out of the house, dribbling a trail of blood behind them. Her head was hanging back and a thin ponytail of fine, soft, straight brown hair fell back from a her small face, her mouth open in a gasping, round "O" … except she wasn't gasping. Her breaths were short and silent.

We put her on the pram and got her into the back of the ambulance as I spiked a bag of saline with a blood pump. Two firemen hopped in the back to ride with my partner, and I jumped in front to drive emergent to Longmont United. As I drove, over the sound of the siren, I heard a loud, guttural groan — the sound made by a sedated animal who would be angry if not for the drug-induced lethargy. My partner was putting a tube down her throat to breathe for her while one firefighter placed defibrillator patches on her chest in case her heart stopped beating, and the other firefighter tried unsuccessfully to start an IV and give her fluids.

At the hospital, we ran the patient inside with the heart monitor propped on her knees. There was a flurry of activity as hospital staff ran to meet us at the doors and move her over into their bed. A dozen hands reached for her and cut off her clothes revealing a slight, undeveloped body, too thin. Too thin. Unfinished like her unfinished life, skin so pale, like skim milk, bones so tiny and protruding. Toes with chipped, dark red nail polish becoming a sickly grey-green-blue color. IVs were started, chest films ordered, a catheter placed. While this happened, the E.R. doctor went into a quiet room with the girl's family and told them what was going on. After a few moments, he came back into the trauma room just as a nurse began to infuse the first unit of blood.

"Stop," he said.

Everyone in the room looked at him, startled, their hands still moving, doing what they were doing, unsure if they had heard correctly and there was not a moment to lose. The nurse froze, face jerking in the direction of the doctor as she squeezed the bag of blood between her hands.

"Her mom wants us to stop." His voice was matter of fact, devoid of emotion — disappointment, disapproval, sadness, anger.

"She doesn't want the organs to be donated, and she knows the patient cannot survive or recover from these injuries, so she wants us to just let her go. Let's get the body cleaned up. The family will be coming in to view her momentarily."

He might have been saying, "Let's get some IVs started and

give her some fluid," but his face was tired, let down. We are here to do what we can until a life is lost beyond recovery.

To simply let a life go is difficult. It goes against our nature. The shoulders of everyone in the trauma room slumped and many eyes turned toward the monitor, where the green, zigzagging line of peaks and valleys proclaimed that the girl still had a beating heart. The sound of rushing air stopped as the person squeezing the bag that filled the patient's lungs with oxygen released it one last time and stepped back. The waves of the girl's heartbeat peaked slower.

I did not wait around to watch it stop.

Outside I cleaned our bloody backboard with disinfectant wipes. She had not bled that much, considering what she had done. Not like the middle aged man who had similarly shot himself a year ago and left our ambulance a war zone. This was a small, tidy mess.

Small.

The girl had not, could not, have completed all that she was meant to with her life. Even in death, what remains behind will not fulfill a greater purpose.

The girl was undone, the day she died.

She was 15 years old.

Chapter 30

First Bad Call

By Jesi Block

I am a third-generation EMT. My grandfather and father were both EMTs on the fire department in the town where I was raised. I had been working retail for a few years. I was bored with it and needed a change. I knew my dad and grandpa had loved being EMTs on the fire department, so I decided to go to school and see if I could get a job working on an ambulance.

The first several weeks of working on the streets as an EMT on an ACLS (advanced cardiac life support) ambulance, I went home crying every day. I was stressed out to the max and feeling afraid. Even though I was a National Registry-certified EMT, I didn't feel like I knew what the heck I was doing. What had I been thinking? Why hadn't I just stayed in retail? Retail eats your soul, but at least lives aren't at stake. But I had quit my job in retail, I had been hired at a private ambulance service, and now here I was scared out of my mind.

It probably took a good three months before I started to get a handle on things. After I had gotten semi-comfortable on the streets, I was assigned a paramedic partner who had been in the field for close to a decade. Nothing fazed her. If I could describe her in one word, it would be "inspirational." She seemed to be in total control of everything that was going on. After we completed calls, we would talk about them, and she would ask me if I had noticed the cigarette that was still lit in the ashtray at the home of the woman who had difficulty breathing or if I had seen the bottle of vodka tucked in the couch cushion at the home of the man who had been throwing up blood for the past 12 hours. Of course, I hadn't seen any of those things. I wondered if I would ever be able to catch all those little things that can really explain what is going on with the patient.

I had been working with Kris for a few weeks and was really enjoying learning all I could from her. On the last shift on our rotation, we asked to be called in early so Kris could catch a flight to Phoenix for the Fourth of July to be with her boyfriend and his family. I was their ride to the airport. We were about 10 minutes away from being called off when a call dropped. Darn it — we had to get to the airport, but we were the only ambulance for the city. The call came across as an auto vs. pedestrian. These calls are usually in reference to accidents that happen at very low speeds, thus causing very minor injuries, sometimes none at all. We were so close to the call that by the time we arrived, the reporting party was still on the phone with the dispatcher.

When we got to the scene, a bystander was waving me down. I pulled the ambulance right next to the patient. I looked out of my window and saw a man in his late 20s lying under a car. He was missing his right lower leg. My partner, knowing how new I was, placed her hand on my forearm and said, "Jesi, he's dead." Now instead of a simple low-speed, non-injury accident, we were dealing with a person who was pinned under a car, unconscious, not breathing. The fire engine that was a few minutes behind us called in another engine for extrication (specialized tools used for getting patients that are trapped in cars).

Kris got out of the ambulance and started assessing the man on the ground. She directed me to the driver of the car — the less critical patient — and told me to check her out. She had a little facial trauma from the airbag that had been deployed and hit her in the face. She was oriented to person, place, time and event but seemed a little slow to respond. She said that she was worried about her husband who she was going to pick up at the bus stop and he was waiting for her, so she didn't want to go to the hospital. I told her that skipping a trip to the hospital wasn't an option and that I was going to call a second ambulance for her. She reluctantly agreed.

By this time, the other fire engines were starting to arrive. I looked for my partner. Where was she? The person who had called 911 said the man wasn't conscious, wasn't breathing, and Kris had told me as soon as we arrived that the patient was dead, so maybe she was just doing what she needed to do for a field pronouncement.

But suddenly, Kris was at my side, asking me for a backboard and C-collars.

I couldn't believe it. He was alive. We were working him.

The scramble on scene began. Four cop cars, two fire engines, two ambulances, all to take care of this one man and the woman who hit him. Not to mention the tons of neighbors, the press, who were all watching what was going on. I can do this, I told myself. I went to the back, started to spike two blood pumps (IVs that can deliver a lot of fluid or blood in a short time) and got some other supplies out for controlling his airway. In the amount of time it took me to do this, my partner had the scene coordinated.

The patient was collared and on a backboard, and CPR was in progress.

"Kris," I asked, "What do you need?"

"I've got it," Kris said. "Let's go." She jumped into the back of the ambulance with two firefighters.

Just as we were about to pull out, the patient's wife showed up. She was frantic, in my way.

"We were just married yesterday," she sobbed hysterically. "I have to go with him."

She wanted to know if she could come in the ambulance with me. Absolutely not, I said. I knew Kris would never allow that. Anxious family hinders the care we provide the patient. Inside I'm reeling. This might be the last time she would see her husband at their new home.

I drove us all to the hospital emergent.

"Slow down!" Kris yelled forward to me. "We have to get some work done."

I did as she asked, but it's hard to remain calm when there is some guy dying in the back of your vehicle. I took a deep breath and tried to suck the tears back into my eyes. It felt just like being a new EMT again.

We dropped him off at the hospital to a team of people that had their focus on just him. "He'll be OK, right?" I asked in the back of my mind. "It's just an amputation," I tried to tell myself.

After dropping the patient at the hospital, we cleaned up the ambulance and took off for our base. My partner still had a plane to catch. Life goes on, at least for some people. On the way to the airport, Kris and I talked about the call. She said I had done a good job, even with driving a little fast. I was feeling better.

I called the hospital a few times after I dropped Kris and her boyfriend off at the airport. His injuries were more extensive than I knew. He had suffered a fracture to the back of his skull. During the night, the surgeons amputated his leg below the knee, and he was under constant supervision because of the pressure on his brain.

When I woke up the next morning, I called again for a patient update.

I couldn't believe my ears.

They were harvesting his organs. He was 28 years old. He had been married the day before. He had been getting his wedding presents out of his car when a woman driving under the influence of prescription drugs hit him. The woman could have crashed anywhere else along the street, and all she would have done was wrecked her car and banged up her face.

It's back to work tomorrow. I picked up a shift to help pay the bills. Wonder what calls I'll go on tomorrow?

Chapter 31

And then there was that one day ...

By Lana Bond

Some days are truly epic. Yesterday I picked up a shift on my day off thinking I would be working with my roommate. Turned out he was working late the night before and chose not to come in, so I ended up working with a part-time medic who picks up a shift, oh, maybe once a year. Goody. That was my first hint that the day would be, well, epic.

I hopped into the ambulance, checked everything out (pretty darn thoroughly) and got ready to begin the day. I was hoping for an interesting medical call, and was getting a strong feeling that we might run a cardiac arrest or something equally intense. Glancing up, I realized that it had gotten cloudy and hazy out, and that the air had that heavy, damp feeling it gets before it begins to (you guessed it) snow! Large, wet, white flakes began to plummet down, turning the streets into a large, wet, white skating rink so fast that the cars on the road didn't even have time to slow down (apparently) to a safer speed and began to roll over into ditches or run into other cars or slide off into medians and what have you.

So, after briefly considering breakfast, my partner and I took off on the first of many canceled calls for the day, a medical call. As we headed gingerly out, our dispatcher informed the world that we were on emergency driving policy. Visibility was nothing and the roads were slick and slushy. Cars couldn't see us until we were right behind them, and then they were afraid to pull over or stop quickly for fear they get stuck, or lose control or whatever was running through their brains. Most people managed, and we crept our way along the highway wailing and flashing, until a small blue car in front of us came to a complete stop in the left lane and staunchly refused to pull to the right. No room in the median to the left. My partner stopped the ambulance while we checked to make sure the right lane was clear before we tried to pass him and then we felt a sudden thump from behind. The muscles in my neck tightened and for a second I couldn't decide if we'd hit something or if something had hit us. I hopped out of the ambulance, keeping a sharp eye out for the cars skidding by in the left lane, none of whom stopped to check on the ambulance who had just been rear-ended, or the red jeep Cherokee who had rear-ended the ambulance. The driver of the blue car took off. The driver of the jeep was horrified. We stood on the side of the road as snow gathered on our strobes, and waited for our team leader (supervisor) to come out and take pictures of the damage (minor to both vehicles) get the other driver's info and put us back in service. Meanwhile, another ambulance took our medical call and ran the patient back emergent to the hospital and we got wet hair and cold toes!

On a side note, the other driver really lucked out. If the police department had shown up on this accident she would have been nailed with multiple citations for hitting an emergency vehicle while it was running lights and sirens. Last time someone slid into us on the ice (and we weren't running emergent) the other driver got five tickets.

After finally getting everything straightened out, we crawled, dripping wet and cold, into our ambulance. Cranking the heat, we headed dejectedly back into town with a brand-sparkling-new stack of forms and reports to fill out. We had just barely made it into the city limits when we got sent on an accident. We were halfway up Flag

Road, which is steep and windy, when our dispatchers informed us that the call we were on and the call another one of our other ambulances was on in Creek Canyon were the same call, and that the accident was in the canyon. We turned around and skied our way back down the mountain, meanwhile discovering that our ambulance didn't have chains or "on spots" (automatic chains that drop down under the tires).

From there we proceeded to be sent on, and canceled from, four more accidents. When we finally made it to one of the accidents we were dispatched to, we found an 18-year-old girl, car nosed into a traffic light pole, sitting in the driver's seat of her car with a C-collar around her neck and fire holding her head on. She was crying, naturally. I jogged over and said, "Hi! I'm Lana. What happened?"

"I was stopping for the light and my car slid on the ice into the light pole. I wasn't going very fast, but my airbags went off in my face and scared me ... "

"Does your neck hurt?"

"No ... "

Why does she have a collar on??? Sigh.

The rule is that if the patient has on a collar we have to immobilize them on a backboard and take them to the hospital. Technically, we are not allowed to take the collar off — only the hospital can. If I'd been working with just about anyone else I would have ignored that rule, taken the collar off and headed on my merry way. She didn't need to go to the hospital. But I wasn't going to take any chances with my partner for the day. Besides, the fire people would have gotten upset if I had usurped their authority and then there would have been meetings and all that. I ran back to the ambulance for the pram and the board (which both promptly became soaked with snow) and suddenly it occurred to me, where was my partner? I peeked around the ambulance and saw she was only just getting out of the ambulance. Sigh.

Then I turned around to find that the firefighter who had been holding the patient's head had wandered off and that the patient was sitting in the car with the collar on alone. (The rule is, if you grab someone's head on a scene you are *married* to it from that point until the patient is fully immobilized. You can not let go!!!)

"Hey. You. Grab her head please!"

Huff. Eyes rolling. Hey, *you started it!*

We get our patient boarded. We get her into the ambulance. I look at my partner, who was doing — I'm not sure what for this whole process— and I was wet and I was grouchy and this was definitely a BLS (basic life support) patient, but what the hell, I was so frustrated and my partner doesn't know the protocol anyway ...

"She's all yours. We don't know if she lost consciousness or not," I say to the part-time paramedic.

We are off on our merry way after giving fire props for helping out. By this point I was actually glad we were taking someone to the hospital whether she needed it or not, since going to Community Hospital meant that I would be near a bathroom. I had needed to pee for the last hour but never got a chance since we kept going on cancellations!

So we're heading up Broadway toward the hospital when another call drops, about three blocks away from us, for chest pain. I glance back. I hear that the only person left available for the call is our team leader, who can't transport because he works alone.

"Um. Five (our radio designation). Our current patient is not emergent. We can take that call if you need and double load ... "

"Five, I have you going to the call. Twenty (the team leader's radio designation) stay in service."

We wail our way to the second call and promptly discover that we can't find the entrance. Anywhere. The map book is no help. Our dispatcher can't help. We finally find our way in almost by accident, and we are ushered through the gate and find our police escort who is so amped up that he sped off, leaving me creeping with the patient and my partner in the back, through the slush. Finally I stopped at an intersection to wait for our escort to come back for us. By the time we finally made it to the door, our response time was nearly 15 minutes.

So my partner ran in with the kit, monitor and bed while I stayed with the current patient and crossed my fingers, hoping I wasn't missing out on a cardiac alert or, better yet, a cardiac arrest.

Our second patient came out to the ambulance with a plethora of wires in tow. He seemed pretty chipper for a guy who'd been in SVT (supra-ventricular tachycardia) when my partner showed up and was now throwing PVC's every fourth or fifth beat.

Having helped load patient No. 2 and started an IV on him, I hopped back in the front to take patient No. 1, patient No. 2, my partner (and a partridge in a pear tree) to Community Hospital. On my way there I thought to myself, "Whew... no more stops, I hope!"

As I pulled up the intersection at First and Broadway I gave myself a good amount of braking space to make sure I had plenty of time to come to a full stop at the light. Just before I came to a complete stop (tires pointing straight ahead), I felt my ambulance begin to drift right at what felt like about 100 miles per hour (though I was barely moving). I believe the sound I made went something like "sssshhhhhhhiiiiiiiiiiiiiiii..........t!!!!" I couldn't turn the tires into the skid because that would turn us into the side of the car next to us, so I jerked the wheel left and then back right. Our ambulance came to rest about one inch away from the driver's side front door of a gold-colored, four-door sedan. I glanced under my eyelashes at the car next to me and found five blue-haired senior citizens staring saucer-eyed at the ambulance that had nearly hit them.

"*Ttsaaaahhhh ...* " hissed between my teeth while the load in the back of my ambulance listened.

"I'd like to know where all our gravel and salt trucks are right now!!!"

(I later found out that our chest-painer was a city councilman. Errr ...)

We dropped our patient's off and turned to our massive stack of paperwork. A blessed five minutes of peace and ...

"Fire and ambulance respond to the rec center for a possible suicide. Our RP (reporting party) states the patient may have tried to commit suicide by drowning himself in the jacuzzi. It is estimated that he spent about six minutes under water."

We showed on scene to find fire holding a large man on his side, back facing us with a puddle of blood under his head. They were suctioning blood out of his mouth. He was looking a bit gray, our guy was. We rolled him onto his back and saw that his mouth was a mass of red and that he had an OPA (oral pharyngeal airway) between his teeth. As we rolled him a woman called to us, "He has epilepsy!"

I nodded.

"Ah," I thought to myself. "He had a seizure in the hot tub. He's postictal. This guy isn't a drowning patient, he's a seizure patient!" People usually don't breathe while they're seizing. Even if he had spent the duration of his seizure with his head under the water the likelihood that he breathed a significant amount of it into his lungs (aspiration) is pretty small. Plus, that would explain the blood. Maybe he bit his tongue.

I looked at my partner. She nodded. And proceeded to treat the patient as a drowning victim. The patient had what I think was another seizure. She thought he was choking on the OPA and had someone pull it out. I went to get a line on him. My partner tried to nasally intubate him (put a tube down his nose into his lungs to breathe for him). I'm not sure why. He was already breathing. Which gave him a bloody nose. Which he promptly began to aspirate. It also pissed him off enough that he began to flail and pulled his IV out. I threw the bloody catheter aside and looked up to see a fire EMT with a BVM (bag valve mask) out trying to securely seal the mask over the patient's cheek while she eagerly bagged the side of his head.

"Your mask has slipped."

"I know that. I'm trying."

"Here. Give me that."

By now the patient was taking rapid, gasping breaths in and out of his mouth, spraying bloody fluid through his lips and into the air. I grabbed the mask and the patient's jaw with both hands, did a jaw thrust while I mashed the plastic to his face, and grabbed the only bystander with gloves on.

"You in the white shirt! Come squeeze this bag!"

The pool lifeguard came over and was so amped that he began to ventilate the patient with about 30 breaths per minute. Hmm. Twenty would be quite sufficient.

"OK. I need you to slow way down. Squeeze the bag in for a slow count of five and then let go. Got that?" He nodded and slowed down the respirations while I continued trying to maintain a seal over the patient's face, now slippery with blood and other fluids. And the patient began to flail and shake his head violently again. The onslaught of gooey red continued to fly threw the air. Finally, my partner made the decision to transport. (I still don't know what she was doing the whole time I was giving the first responder/life guard his bagging and ventilation lesson.) We began the process of wheeling the patient out through the men's locker room and out to the ambulance with my partner (actually doing something), a firefighter holding the mask, me bagging, and another firefighter all in tow. I had just enough time to throw a quick thank you over my shoulder to the first responder and we were out in the snow and back into the overheated back of our ambulance. My partner grabbed two firefighters to ride in the back and I hopped into the front after peeling off my gooey gloves and discovering that I had a fresh, open cut on the back of my hand. My hand was red, and I didn't know if it was all my blood or if some of his had seeped into my glove.

We wailed and flashed our way to the hospital. The transport was just long enough for my partner and our two riders to touch *everything* in the back of the ambulance at least once with their bloody, bloody hands. They never got a tube. They never got a successful line. They never figured out that this patient needed valium and an oral tube.

They suctioned.

We pulled into the bay, I gloved up and we unloaded. At the hospital, they sedated our guy with Ativan and tubed him. They hooked him up to a respirator. They flushed out his lungs with saline. They didn't use fresh water because it is hypotonic (That means it has a lower sodium content than the fluid in your cells and will draw water out of the cells of your lungs if you aspirate it.) They sent him to CT for a CAT scan.

I went into the bathroom to look at myself. My face and arms were splattered with blood. My white shirt looked like I had made spaghetti sauce at work. My pants had rusty drips and drizzles all down the front. I looked down at my bloody self and thought to myself, "What if he has HIV?" I felt myself choke.

So we stayed at the hospital, my partner and I, for three hours while I cleaned up the back of our ambulance. Texas chainsaw massacre, I kid you not. There was not a single surface that had not been sprayed with blood. Even after we wiped everything down and cleaned and stocked the kit, and cleaned and stocked the monitor, and cleaned and re-sheeted the pram, the cabinets of the ambulance bled the patient's blood until the end of our shift. We went through prophylactic exposure procedures, where they draw his blood and then draw our blood. They test us. We fill out piles of forms.

While we finished up at the hospital another one of our crews came in with a CPR in progress. I opened their back door to see a surprisingly young female with her chest being pumped and an oral tube being successfully placed. Then the medic vented the patient's chest by sticking a large needle between her ribs and into her chest cavity to re-inflate a collapsed lung. The patient was finally pronounced dead in the hospital just a few minutes later. She had a collapsed valve in her heart and had dropped dead at the grocery store where she worked. She was only 27.

I helped that crew put their ambulance back together.

Our dispatcher called us out of service for the day and we headed back to ops, our base. On the way in, I noticed that the snow had finally stopped.

We got back to the station three hours before the end of our shift. We spent that three hours filling out piles of forms

153

from the day. An accident report and an incident report for the accident. An incident report for the exposure. Plus trip reports for every cancellation and call still left from the day.

As we finally finished up and were getting ready to get the heck out of Dodge, the crew we'd seen at the hospital pulled in looking as bedraggled and mentally and physically exhausted as my partner and I were.

"Hey, you know that guy you brought in from the rec center?"

"Yeah..."

"He died."

"Oooohhhhhh!" Is right.

We didn't run a cardiac arrest yesterday, but we certainly got that interesting medical call I felt we'd have.

On the positive side, I got to see someone's chest successfully vented, and the respiratory therapist at the hospital let me watch him flush our patient's lungs. He had a suction unit attached to a small camera so he could see where the tube was going. There was a port on the side where he could push saline into the tube, and a small canister on the other side to catch the bloody fluid rinsed out of the patient's lungs. He let me look into the camera and see the trachea, the carina, the place where the trachea branches into the bronchioles, and the inside of the patient's lungs. Way cool!

Plus I got to see that I can keep my cool on disastrous scenes, even if everyone else (including my partner) is panicking.

I also got to see that my instincts are sometimes really good, and that I should be more aggressive about voicing them. If I had, that guy might not have gotten the bloody nose from the nasal tube and maybe wouldn't have breathed in so much fluid. I think he would have died anyway, but at least I wouldn't feel like we sped up the process.

There is always a challenge between voicing my thoughts and causing a disruption on scene by disagreeing with my partner.

I got to assert some authority, and I got to create some bonds with some firefighters, some hospital staff, and some patients. That's good.

The day seemed bad right after it was over, because I was physically and emotionally wrecked. But when I think about it, this is what I signed up for. This is what I was hoping for every day when I got into this job. These are the kinds of calls I love. But I love them better when they go well and everything flows the way it should. These are the calls I love when I work with a medic whose judgment I trust and who trusts me enough to hear my opinion and who listens to the other voices on the scene — not just the one inside their head that is giving them tunnel vision.

I love my job. It really is great. But I love it better when we save the people we pick up.

Chapter 32

Radio Report

Paramedic One: "Hospital ER, Paramedic One."

ER: "Go ahead, Paramedic One."

Paramedic One: "We are responding non-emergent with a 49-year-old male. He is an alcoholic and today he told 911 that he was having a heart attack. He has not given us any information and will not give a chief complaint. His EKG looks normal and vitals are within normal limits. He has been to your facility a number of times. We should be there in about five minutes."

ER: "Copy, Paramedic One. Did you bring his wheelchair?"

Paramedic One: "Affirmative."

Chapter 33

The Quotable Joe S. and others

Life should not be journey to the grave with the intention of arriving safely in an attractive and well preserved body, but rather to skid in sideways, chocolate in one hand, martini in the other, body thoroughly used up, totally worn out and screaming, "Woo hoo! What a ride!"
  - Quote found on the refrigerator of a patient

"He wasn't dead, he just smelled like it."
  - Joe S.

"Milk expires. People die."
  - Joe S.

"It's better to be warm and drunk in the Caribbean than cold and dead in Colorado."
  - Joe S.

"Keep her pheromones for the sick and twisted off of me."
  - Joe S.

"I can't make your pain go away instantaneously. This isn't 'Bewitched'".
  - Joe S.

"I've been groped by this patient more in the past 30 minutes than by my husband in a year."
  -Joe S.

"Joe is really good with kids."
>   - Stephanie to concerned mother

"Your crying does not affect me. If you don't stop, I am going to tie you down."
>   - Joe talking to the 12 year old spawn of Satan in the back of the ambulance.

"Please stop trying to make things better. I just want to be upset and cranky."
>   - Joe S.

"You need an interpreter? Stephanie speaks vaginal Spanish!"
>   - Joe S.

"He felt like a cured ham."
>   - Joe referring to a 5-day-old dead body found in a house reeking of cigarette smoke

"You stupid whore."
>   - Joe referring to bad drivers

"Do you have a comb?" - Maxine (age 92)
"No Ma'am, this is an emergency room" - ER nurse
"Then do you have an emergency comb?" - Maxine

"We are not allowed to lift patients."
>   - nurse in a nursing home.

"They have a disease." – Nurse
"Where?" – Joe
"All over." – Nurse

"The patient doesn't know they are being moved to Assisted Living." – Nurse
"Who will tell them?" – Joe
"Their family." – Nurse
"Where is their family?" – Joe
"Oh, they don't have any family." – Nurse

"Sometimes 12 hours just doesn't seem long enough."
    - Stephanie

Others ...

"I'm not afraid of death. I just don't want to be there when it happens."
    - Liz (age 89)

"We are experts at breathing for other people. That is what we do."
    -Will D.

"My entire EMS career is based on eliminating puke."
    -Will D.

"It is hard for the patient to tell the difference between acting brave and being brave."
    -Will D.

"There is an inverse relationship between teeth and tattoos."
    -Will D.

"If it is going to make me puke, I cover it up."
    -Will D.

"Anytime the body suffers an insult, it responds by saying, 'Everybody out! Both exits! No waiting!!'"
    -Will D.

"If you are ever confused in EMS, oxygenate and transport."
     -Will D.

"Don't say 'oops', say 'there.'"
     -Thom D.

"Any word with two u's in it grosses me out. For example, mucus and sputum."
     -Will D.

"Purkinje fibers are the 'Hail Mary' of cardiac function."
     -Will D.

"One of the first rules of EMS: The bigger the person, the smaller the room you will find them in."
     - Will D.

"When I have a band, it will be called Frothy Pink Sputum."
     -Will D.

"The difference between a good and an adequate EMT? The good EMT will eliminate the guesswork."

"Aspirin ain't gonna do dick without the chain of survival."
     -Will D.

"Is your patient dead or deader than hell?"
     -Will D.

"There is nothing worse than sitting in an ambulance, waiting for your patient to land." (Skydiving accident)
     -Will D.

"She was really fucked up. That is a technical term."
     -Thom D.

"Epi dumps are common. I make my partner walk around the ambulance one time before we go inside to a call."
-Will D.

"You're only as good as your last call."
– Jim M.

And more…

"Never lie to your patient. But you don't have to tell them the whole truth either."

"If your patient is sweating, you should be too."

"Remember, you are often seeing people on the worst day of their lives."

"In a real emergency, the best treatment is LSPOR — long skinny pedal on right."

"If you align a bone and still don't have a pulse, it sucks ... but that is why we drive fast."

"Saving lives, making a difference."

"I don't get paid enough to clean toilets."

"No one gets out of this game alive."

"No harm, no foul."

"It seems that every cliché will come true in this job."

DRT — Dead Right There

ABCs- Arrival, Bewilderment, Chopper Go

Dispatch: "Paramedic 1 respond to a code '0' male."
Paramedic One: "Communication, what's a code '0' male?"
Dispatch: "Kind of like your husband, but with glasses."
(This was meant as a joke!)

"Back in the day I was a hymen breaker." Old man answering what he use to do for a living.

"Jesse, grab me a razor for this lady's 12-lead."

"The patient is unconscious, but(t) breathing."

Dispatch: "Paramedic One, respond to a drunk female at Ninth and Main. Somebody is calling on your sister again."
(Call for a frequent flyer, a person who calls 911 a lot).
Paramedic: "You're the one who married her".
(Both the dispatcher and paramedic were having fun).

"Slow down, it's not my emergency." Paramedic to new EMT.

"If by heat emergency you mean vodka-related emergency, yeah it is." – Paramedic to newspaper reporter.

87-year-old patient: "Why are you yelling, I'm not deaf."
38-year-old deaf paramedic: "Well I am."

"Paramedics save lives, EMTs save paramedic's lives."

"Saving lives and living the dream."